**Third Edition
Revised
Reprint**

Certified Coding Associate (CCA) Exam Preparation

Dorine L. Bennett,
EdD, MBA, RHIA, FAHIMA

and

Kathy L. Dorale,
RHIA, CCS, CCS–P

Editors

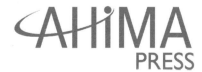

PRESS

ISBN: 978-1-58426-059-2

AHIMA Product No.: AC400313

AHIMA Staff:
Jessica Block, MA, Assistant Editor
Angie Comfort, RHIT, CCS, Technical Review
Katie Greenock, MS, Production Development Editor
Jason O. Malley, Director, Creative Content Development
Pamela Woolf, Managing Editor

For more information, including updates, about AHIMA Press publications, visit http://www.ahima.org/publications/updates.aspx

American Health Information Management Association
233 North Michigan Avenue, 21st Floor
Chicago, Illinois 60601-5809
ahima.org

Contents

Online Assessment

Practice Questions with Answers

Practice Exam 1 with Answers

Practice Exam 2 with Answers

Practice Exam 3 with Answers—*Bonus Exam*

About the Editors

Dorine L. Bennett, EdD, MBA, RHIA, FAHIMA is associate professor and director of the health information management (HIM) programs at Dakota State University (DSU). Before joining the faculty at DSU, Dorine worked in the HIM field in settings such as an acute care hospital, a community health office, and a long-term care system as well as independently contracting as a workshop instructor and consultant for long-term care facilities and acute care and specialty hospitals.

Dorine has completed her undergraduate degrees in health information technology (AS) and health information administration (BS) and earned a master of business administration degree with an emphasis in management of information systems (MBA). She recently earned her doctorate degree in educational administration in adult and higher education.

She has served on a number of committees for the American Health Information Management Association and chaired the AHIMA Fellowship Review Committee. Dorine has been president and director of education for the South Dakota Health Information Management Association, as well as leading and serving on a number of committees for the state association. She is also an accreditation site reviewer for the Commission on Accreditation for Health Informatics and Information Management Education (CAHIIM).

Kathy L. Dorale, RHIA, CCS, CCS-P is the vice president of HIM at Avera Health in Sioux Falls, South Dakota. Kathy provides coding and billing reviews and education for Avera Health's 30 hospitals and multifacility healthcare settings in a five-state region. She has experience working with electronic medical records and revenue cycle initiatives collaboratively with Avera Hospitals. Before working at Avera's corporate office, Kathy was the director of HIM, business office and registration areas, in acute care hospital settings with experience in contract work for long-term care.

Kathy has completed her undergraduate degree in health information administration (BS) and plans to pursue a master's of science in health informatics at Dakota State University.

She has also served as president and treasurer for the South Dakota Health Information Management Association, as well as serving on several committees for the state association. She enjoys speaking engagements on coding and reimbursement topics to affiliated local and state associations and guest speaking for Dakota State University. She also serves on the Provider Roundtable committee with providers across the states. The committee provides comment and testimony on reimbursement and coding issues to the Centers for Medicare and Medicaid–appointed task force during open comment period for the outpatient perspective payment system, biannually, on behalf of all providers.

About the CCA Exam

The certified coding associate (CCA) distinguishes coders by exhibiting commitment and demonstrating coding competencies across all settings, including both hospitals and physician practices. On the basis of job analysis standards and state-of-the-art test construction, the CCA is creating a larger pool of qualified coders ready to meet potential employers' needs. The CCA designation has been a nationally accepted standard of achievement in the health information management (HIM) field since 2002 and is the only HIM credential worldwide currently accredited by the National Commission for Certifying Agencies (NCCA).

Detailed information about the CCA exam including academic eligibility requirements, frequently asked questions, and an exam application can be found at http://ahima.org/certification.

Exam Competency Statements

The CCA certification exam is based on an explicit set of competencies. These competencies have been determined through a job analysis study of practitioners. The competencies are subdivided into domains and tasks, as listed here. The exam tests only content pertaining to these competencies. Each domain is allocated a predefined number of questions at specific cognitive levels to make up the exam.

Domain I: Clinical Classification Systems (32% of Exam)

1. Interpret healthcare data for code assignment
2. Incorporate clinical vocabularies and terminologies used in health information systems
3. Abstract pertinent information from medical records
4. Consult reference materials to facilitate code assignment
5. Apply inpatient coding guidelines
6. Apply outpatient coding guidelines
7. Apply physician coding guidelines
8. Assign inpatient codes
9. Assign outpatient codes
10. Assign physician codes
11. Sequence codes according to healthcare setting

Domain II: Reimbursement Methodologies (23% of Exam)

1. Sequence codes for optimal reimbursement
2. Link diagnoses and CPT codes according to payer specific guidelines
3. Assign correct diagnosis-related group (DRG)
4. Assign correct ambulatory payment classification (APC)
5. Evaluate NCCI (National Correct Coding Initiative) edits
6. Reconcile NCCI edits
7. Validate medical necessity using LCDs (local coverage determinations) and NCDs (national coverage determinations)
8. Submit claim forms
9. Communicate with financial departments
10. Evaluate claim denials

11. Respond to claim denials
12. Resubmit denied claim to the payer source
13. Communicate with the physician to clarify documentation

Domain III: Health Records and Data Content (15% of Exam)

1. Retrieve medical records
2. Assemble medical records according to healthcare setting
3. Analyze medical records quantitatively for completeness
4. Analyze medical records qualitatively for deficiencies
5. Perform data abstraction
6. Request patient-specific documentation from other sources (for example, ancillary departments, physician's office)
7. Retrieve patient information from master patient index
8. Educate providers in regard to health data standards
9. Generate reports for data analysis

Domain IV: Compliance (14% of Exam)

1. Identify discrepancies between coded data and supporting documentation
2. Validate that codes assigned by provider or electronic systems are supported by proper documentation
3. Perform ethical coding
4. Clarify documentation through physician query
5. Research latest coding changes
6. Implement latest coding changes
7. Update fee/charge ticket based on latest coding changes
8. Educate providers on compliant coding
9. Assist in preparing the organization for external audits

Domain V: Information Technologies (8% of Exam)

1. Navigate throughout the electronic health record (EHR)
2. Utilize encoding and grouping software
3. Utilize practice management and HIM systems
4. Utilize computer-assisted coding (CAC) software that automatically assigns codes based on electronic text
5. Validate the codes assigned by CAC software

Domain VI: Confidentiality and Privacy (8% of Exam)

1. Ensure patient confidentiality
2. Educate healthcare staff on privacy and confidentiality issues
3. Recognize and report privacy issues/violations
4. Maintain a secure work environment
5. Utilize pass codes
6. Access only minimal necessary documents/information
7. Release patient-specific data to authorized individuals

8. Protect electronic documents through encryption
9. Transfer electronic documents through secure sites
10. Retain confidential records appropriately
11. Destroy confidential records appropriately

Exam Specifications

The CCA exam consists of 100 multiple choice questions. Candidates have two hours to complete the exam.

For exams scheduled on or after April 1, 2013, the CCA exam is based on ICD-9-CM codes effective October 1, 2011, or October 1, 2012, and CPT codes effective January 1, 2013. All candidates will have to present either the 2012 or 2013 version of the ICD-9 and the 2013 edition of the AMA CPT codebooks in order to test on or after April 1, 2013. If a candidate presents the incorrect codebooks at the testing center, he or she will be turned away and will forfeit the testing fee. For a complete listing of allowable codebooks, visit http://ahima.org/certification.

The Commission on Certification for Health Informatics and Information Management (CCHIIM) manages and sets the strategic direction for the certifications. Pearson Vue is the exclusive provider of AHIMA certification exams. To see sample questions and images of the new exam format, visit http://ahima.org/certification.

How to Use This Book and Online Assessment

The CCA practice questions and practice exams in this book and on the accompanying online assessment test knowledge of content pertaining to the CCA competencies published by AHIMA. The 500 multiple choice questions in this book and online assessment are presented in a similar format to those that might be found on the CCA exam.

This book contains 200 multiple choice practice questions and two multiple choice practice exams (with 100 questions each). In addition, six inpatient and ambulatory coding cases have been added to the practice questions in this reprint. Because each question is identified with one of the six CCA domains, you will be able to determine whether you need knowledge or skill building in particular areas of the exam. Most questions provide an answer rationale and reference. Pursuing the sources of these references will help build your knowledge and skills.

To most effectively use this book, work through all the practice questions first. This will help identify areas in which you may need further preparation. After going through the practice questions, take one of the practice exams. Again, for the questions that you answer incorrectly, refresh your knowledge by reading the associated references. Continue in the same manner with the second and third practice exams.

The online assessment contains the same 200 practice questions covering all six CCA domains, six practice coding case studies, and two timed practice exams printed in the book, plus a third *bonus* practice exam. These timed, self-scoring exams can be run in practice mode—which allows you to work at your own pace—or exam simulation mode—which simulates the two-hour, timed exam experience. You may retake the practice questions and exams as many times as you like. The practice questions and simulated practice exams online can be set to be presented in random order, or you may choose to go through the questions in sequential order by domain. You may also choose to practice or test your skills on specific domains. For example, if you would like to build your skills in domain 3, you may choose only domain 3 questions for a given practice session.

Acknowledgements

The authors and AHIMA Press would like to acknowledge Jennifer Hornung Garvin, PhD, MBA, RHIA, CCS, CPHQ, CTR, FAHIMA, for contributing the practice question case studies included in this revision.

PRACTICE QUESTIONS

Domain I   *Clinical Classification Systems*

1. Identify the diagnosis code(s) for carcinoma in situ of vocal cord.

   a. 231.0

   b. 161.0

   c. 239.1

   d. 212.1

2. Identify the diagnosis code(s) for melanoma of skin of shoulder.

   a. 172.8, 172.6

   b. 172.6

   c. 172.9

   d. 172.8

3. Which of the following organizations is responsible for updating the procedure classification of ICD-9-CM?

   a. Centers for Disease Control (CDC)

   b. Centers for Medicare and Medicaid Services (CMS)

   c. National Center for Health Statistics (NCHS)

   d. World Health Organization (WHO)

4. At which level of the classification system are the most specific ICD-9-CM codes found?

   a. Category level

   b. Section level

   c. Subcategory level

   d. Subclassification level

5. What are five-digit ICD-9-CM diagnosis codes referred to as?

   a. Category codes

   b. Section codes

   c. Subcategory codes

   d. Subclassification codes

6. What are four-digit ICD-9-CM diagnosis codes referred to as?

   a. Category codes

   b. Section codes

   c. Subcategory codes

   d. Subclassification codes

7. Which of the following ICD-9-CM codes are always alphanumeric?

   a. Category codes

   b. Procedure codes

   c. Subcategory codes

   d. V codes

8. Which of the following ICD-9-CM codes classify environmental events and circumstances as the cause of an injury, poisoning, or other adverse effect?

   a. Category codes

   b. E codes

   c. Subcategory codes

   d. V codes

9. Which volume of ICD-9-CM contains the Tabular and Alphabetic Index of procedures?

   a. Volume 1

   b. Volume 2

   c. Volume 3

   d. Volume 4

10. Identify the correct diagnosis code for lipoma of the face.

    a. 214.1

    b. 213.0

    c. 214.0

    d. 214.9

11. Identify the correct diagnosis code(s) for adenoma of adrenal cortex with Conn's syndrome.

    a. 227.0, 255.12

    b. 227.0

    c. 255.12

    d. 225.12, 227.8

12. Which of the following is a standard terminology used to code medical procedures and services?

    a. CPT

    b. HCPCS

    c. ICD-9-CM

    d. SNOMED CT

13. Identify the appropriate ICD-9-CM diagnosis code for cerebral contusion with brief loss of consciousness.

    a. 924.9

    b. 851.42

    c. 851.82

    d. 851.81

14. If a patient has an excision of a malignant lesion of the skin, the CPT code is determined by the body area from which the excision occurs and which of the following?

    a. Length of the lesion as described in the pathology report

    b. Dimension of the specimen submitted as described in the pathology report

    c. Width times the length of the lesion as described in the operative report

    d. Diameter of the lesion as well as the most narrow margins required to adequately excise the lesion described in the operative report

15. According to CPT, a repair of a laceration that includes retention sutures would be considered what type of closure?

    a. Complex

    b. Intermediate

    c. Not specified

    d. Simple

16. A patient is admitted with spotting. She had been treated two weeks previously for a miscarriage with sepsis. The sepsis had resolved, and she is afebrile at this time. She is treated with an aspiration dilation and curettage. Products of conception are found. Which of the following should be the principal diagnosis?

    a. Miscarriage

    b. Complications of spontaneous abortion with sepsis

    c. Sepsis

    d. Spontaneous abortion with sepsis

17. An 80-year-old female is admitted with fever, lethargy, hypotension, tachycardia, oliguria, and elevated WBC. The patient has more than 100,000 organisms of *Escherichia coli* per cc of urine. The attending physician documents "urosepsis." How should the coder proceed to code this case?

    a. Code sepsis as the principal diagnosis with urinary tract infection due to *E. coli* as secondary diagnosis.

    b. Code urinary tract infection with sepsis as the principal diagnosis.

    c. Query the physician to ask if the patient has septicemia because of the symptomatology.

    d. Query the physician to ask if the patient had septic shock so that this may be used as the principal diagnosis.

18. A 65-year-old patient, with a history of lung cancer, is admitted to a healthcare facility with ataxia and syncope and a fractured arm as a result of falling. The patient undergoes a closed reduction of the fracture in the emergency department and undergoes a complete workup for metastatic carcinoma of the brain. The patient is found to have metastatic carcinoma of the lung to the brain and undergoes radiation therapy to the brain. Which of the following would be the principal diagnosis in this case?

    a. Ataxia

    b. Fractured arm

    c. Metastatic carcinoma of the brain

    d. Carcinoma of the lung

19. A patient was admitted for abdominal pain with diarrhea and was diagnosed with infectious gastroenteritis. The patient also has angina and chronic obstructive pulmonary disease. Which of the following would be the correct coding and sequencing for this case?

    a. Abdominal pain; infectious gastroenteritis; chronic obstructive pulmonary disease; angina

    b. Infectious gastroenteritis; chronic obstructive pulmonary disease; angina

    c. Gastroenteritis; abdominal pain; angina

    d. Gastroenteritis; abdominal pain; diarrhea; chronic obstructive pulmonary disease; angina

20. A patient is admitted with a history of prostate cancer and with mental confusion. The patient completed radiation therapy for prostatic carcinoma three years ago and is status post a radical resection of the prostate. A CT scan of the brain during the current admission reveals metastasis. Which of the following is the correct coding and sequencing for the current hospital stay?

    a. Metastatic carcinoma of the brain; carcinoma of the prostate; mental confusion

    b. Mental confusion; history of carcinoma of the prostate; admission for chemotherapy

    c. Metastatic carcinoma of the brain; history of carcinoma of the prostate

    d. Carcinoma of the prostate; metastatic carcinoma to the brain

21. A patient is admitted with abdominal pain. The physician states that the discharge diagnosis is pancreatitis versus noncalculus cholecystitis. Both diagnoses are equally treated. The correct coding and sequencing for this case would be:

    a. Sequence either the pancreatitis or noncalculus cholecystitis as principal diagnosis

    b. Pancreatitis; noncalculus cholecystitis; abdominal pain

    c. Noncalculus cholecystitis; pancreatitis; abdominal pain

    d. Abdominal pain; pancreatitis; noncalculus cholecystitis

22. According to the UHDDS, which of the following is the definition of "other diagnoses"?

    a. Is recorded in the patient record

    b. Is documented by the attending physician

    c. Receives clinical evaluation or therapeutic treatment or diagnostic procedures or extends the length of stay or increases nursing care and monitoring

    d. Is documented by at least two physicians and the nursing staff

23. A 7-year-old patient was admitted to the emergency department for treatment of shortness of breath. The patient is given epinephrine and nebulizer treatments. The shortness of breath and wheezing are unabated following treatment. What diagnosis should be suspected?

    a. Acute bronchitis

    b. Acute bronchitis with chronic obstructive pulmonary disease

    c. Asthma with status asthmaticus

    d. Chronic obstructive asthma

24. A patient is seen in the emergency department for chest pain. After evaluation of the patient it is suspected that the patient may have gastroesophageal reflux disease (GERD). The final diagnosis was "Rule out chest pain versus GERD." The correct ICD-9-CM code is:

    a. V71.7, Admission for suspected cardiovascular condition

    b. 789.01, Esophageal pain

    c. 530.81, Gastrointestinal reflux

    d. 786.50, Chest pain NOS

25. A skin lesion is removed from a patient's cheek in the dermatologist's office. The dermatologist documents "skin lesion" in the health record. Before billing the pathology report returns with a diagnosis of basal cell carcinoma. Which of the following actions should the coding professional do for claim submission?

    a. Code skin lesion

    b. Code benign skin lesion

    c. Code basal cell carcinoma

    d. Query the dermatologist

26. An epidural was given during labor. Subsequently, it was determined that the patient would require a C-section for cephalopelvic disproportion because of obstructed labor. Assign the correct ICD-9-CM diagnostic and CPT anesthesia codes. (Modifiers are not used in this example.)

    a. 660.11, 653.41, 64479

    b. 660.11, 653.01, 01961

    c. 660.11, 653.41, 01967, 01968

    d. 660.11, 653.91, 01996

27. Which of the following statements does *not* apply to ICD-9-CM?

    a. It can be used as the basis for epidemiological research.

    b. It can be used in the evaluation of medical care planning for healthcare delivery systems.

    c. It can be used to facilitate data storage and retrieval.

    d. It can be used to collect data about nursing care.

28. Which of the following is *not* one of the purposes of ICD-9-CM?

    a. Classification of morbidity for statistical purposes

    b. Classification of mortality for statistical purposes

    c. Reporting of diagnoses by physicians

    d. Identification of the supplies, products, and services provided to patients

29. Which volume of ICD-9-CM contains the numerical listing of codes that represent diseases and injuries?

    a. Volume 1

    b. Volume 2

    c. Volume 3

    d. Volume 4

30. When coding benign neoplasm of the skin, the section noted here directs the coder to:

216	Benign Neoplasm of Skin	
	Includes:	
		Blue Nevus
		Dermatofibroma
		Hydrocystoma
		Pigmented Nevus
		Syringoadenoma
		Syringoma
	Excludes:	
		Skin of genital organs (221.0–222.9)
216.0	Skin of lip	
	Excludes:	
		Vermilion border of lip (210.0)
216.1	Eyelid, including canthus	
	Excludes:	
		Cartilage of eyelid (215.0)

a. Use category 216 for syringoma.

b. Use category 216 for malignant melanoma.

c. Use category 216 for malignant neoplasm of the bone.

d. Use category 216 for malignant neoplasm of the skin.

31. A patient was discharged with the following diagnoses: "Cerebral occlusion, hemiparesis, and hypertension. The aphasia resolved before the patient was discharged." Which of the following code assignments would be appropriate for this case?

342.90	Hemiparesis affecting unspecified side
342.91	Hemiparesis affecting dominant side
342.92	Hemiparesis affecting nondominant side
434.90	Cerebral artery occlusion unspecified, without mention of cerebral infarction
434.91	Cerebral artery occlusion unspecified with cerebral infarction
401	Hypertension
401.0	Malignant hypertension
401.1	Benign hypertension
401.9	Unspecified hypertension
428.0	Congestive heart failure
784.3	Aphasia

a. 434.91, 342.92, 784.3, 401

b. 434.90, 342.90, 784.3, 401.9

c. 434.90, 342.90, 401.9

d. 434.90, 342.90, 784.3, 401.0

32. A patient is admitted to the hospital with shortness of breath and congestive heart failure. The patient subsequently develops respiratory failure. The patient undergoes intubation with ventilator management. Which of the following would be the correct sequencing and coding of this case?

    a. Congestive heart failure, respiratory failure, ventilator management, intubation

    b. Respiratory failure, intubation, ventilator management

    c. Respiratory failure, congestive heart failure, intubation, ventilator management

    d. Shortness of breath, congestive heart failure, respiratory failure, ventilator management

33. A physician correctly prescribes Coumadin. The patient takes the Coumadin as prescribed but develops hematuria as a result of taking the medication. Which of the following is the correct way to code this case?

    a. Poisoning due to Coumadin

    b. Unspecified adverse reaction to Coumadin

    c. Hematuria; poisoning due to Coumadin

    d. Hematuria; adverse reaction to Coumadin

34. A patient is admitted for chest pain with cardiac dysrhythmia to Hospital A. The patient is found to have an acute inferior myocardial infarction with atrial fibrillation. After the atrial fibrillation was controlled and the patient was stabilized, the patient was transferred to Hospital B for a CABG X3. Using the codes listed here, what are the appropriate ICD-9-CM codes and sequencing for both hospitalizations?

410.00	Myocardial infarction of anterolateral wall, episode unspecified
410.01	Myocardial infarction of anterolateral wall, initial episode
410.40	Myocardial infarction of inferior wall, episode unspecified
410.41	Myocardial infarction of inferior wall, initial episode
410.42	Myocardial infarction of inferior wall, subsequent episode
427	Cardiac dysrhythmias
427.3	Atrial fibrillation and flutter
427.31	Atrial fibrillation
786.50	Chest pain, unspecified
36.13	Aortocoronary bypass of three coronary arteries

    a. Hospital A: 427, 786.50, 427.31, 410.91; Hospital B: 410.92, 36.13

    b. Hospital A: 410.41, 427, 427.31; Hospital B: 410.42, 36.13

    c. Hospital A: 410.41, 427.31; Hospital B: 410.41, 36.13

    d. Hospital A: 410.41, 427.31, 786.50; Hospital B: 410.42, 36.13

35. A patient is admitted to the hospital with abdominal pain. The principal diagnosis is cholecystitis. The patient also has a history of hypertension and diabetes. In the DRG prospective payment system, which of the following would determine the MDC assignment for this patient?

    a. Abdominal pain

    b. Cholecystitis

    c. Hypertension

    d. Diabetes

36. A patient was admitted to the hospital with symptoms of a stroke and secondary diagnoses of COPD and hypertension. The patient was subsequently discharged from the hospital with a principal diagnosis of cerebral vascular accident and secondary diagnoses of catheter-associated urinary tract infection, COPD, and hypertension. Which of the following diagnoses should *not* be tagged as POA?

    a. Catheter-associated urinary tract infection

    b. Cerebral vascular accident

    c. COPD

    d. Hypertension

37. Which of the following is a condition that arises during hospitalization?

    a. Case mix

    b. Complication

    c. Comorbidity

    d. Principal diagnosis

38. A 65-year-old female was admitted to the hospital. She was diagnosed with septicemia secondary to *Staphylococcus aureus* and abdominal pain secondary to diverticulitis of the colon. What is the correct code assignment?

    a. 038.8, 562.11, 789.00

    b. 038.11, 562.11

    c. 038.8, 562.11, 041.11

    d. 038.9, 562.11

39. Patient had carcinoma of the anterior bladder wall fulgurated three years ago. The patient returns yearly for a cystoscopy to recheck for bladder tumor. Patient is currently admitted for a routine check. A small recurring malignancy is found and fulgurated during the cystoscopy procedure. Which is the correct code assignment?

    a. 188.3, V10.51, 57.49, 57.32

    b. 198.1, 57.49

    c. 188.3, 57.49

    d. 198.1, 188.3, 57.49

40. A patient with a diagnosis of ventral hernia is admitted to undergo a laparotomy with ventral hernia repair. The patient undergoes a laparotomy and develops bradycardia. The operative site is closed without the repair of the hernia. Which is the correct code assignment?

    a. 553.20, 427.89, V64.3, 54.11

    b. 553.20, 997.1, 427.89, 54.19

    c. 553.20, 54.11

    d. 553.20, 54.11, V64.3

41. These codes are used to assign a diagnosis to a patient who is seeking health services but is not necessarily sick.

    a. E codes

    b. V codes

    c. M codes

    d. C codes

42. Patient was admitted through the emergency department following a fall from a ladder while painting an interior room in his house. He had contusions of the scalp and face and an open fracture of the acetabulum. The fracture site was debrided and the fracture was reduced by open procedure with an external fixation device applied. Which is the correct code assignment?

    a. 808.1, E881.0, E849.0, 79.25, 78.15

    b. 808.1, 920, E881.0, E849.0, E000.8, E013.9, 79.25, 78.15, 79.65

    c. 808.0, E881.0, E000.8, E013.9, 79.35, 79.65

    d. 808.1, E881.0, E849.0, E013.9, 79.25, 78.15, 79.65

43. Assign the correct CPT code for the following procedure: Revision of the pacemaker skin pocket.

    a. 33223

    b. 33210

    c. 33212

    d. 33222

44. Assign the correct CPT code for the following: A 58-year-old male was seen in the outpatient surgical center for an insertion of self-contained inflatable penile prosthesis for impotence.

    a. 54401

    b. 54405

    c. 54440

    d. 54400

45. Patient returns during a 90-day postoperative period from a ventral hernia repair, now complaining of eye pain. What modifier would a physician setting use with the Evaluation and Management code?

    a. −79, Unrelated procedure or service by the same physician during the postoperative period

    b. −25, Significant, separately identifiable evaluation and management service by the same physician on the same day of the procedure or other service

    c. −21, Prolonged evaluation and management services

    d. −24, Unrelated evaluation and management service by the same physician during a postoperative period

46. A patient is admitted to an acute-care hospital for acute intoxication and alcohol withdrawal syndrome due to chronic alcoholism.

    a. 291.8, 303.00

    b. 303.00

    c. 305.00

    d. 291.81, 303.00

47. A 45-year-old female is admitted for blood loss anemia due to dysfunctional uterine bleeding.

    a. 280.0, 626.8

    b. 285.1, 626.8

    c. 626.8, 280.0

    d. 280.0, 218.9

48. Patient admitted with senile cataract, diabetes mellitus, and extracapsular cataract extraction with simultaneous insertion of intraocular lens.

    a. 366.10, 250.50, 13.59, 13.71

    b. 250.00, 366.10

    c. 250.00, 366.12

    d. 366.10, 250.00, 13.59, 13.71

49. A patient is admitted with acute exacerbation of COPD, chronic renal failure, and hypertension.

    a. 492.8, 496, 403.10, 585.9

    b. 492.8, 585.9, 401.9

    c. 496, 585.9, 401.9

    d. 491.21, 403.91, 585.9

50. Patient arrived by ambulance to the emergency department following a motor vehicle accident. Patient sustained a fracture of the ankle; 3.0-cm superficial laceration of the left arm; 5.0-cm laceration of the scalp with exposure of the fascia; and a concussion. Patient received the following procedures: X-ray of the ankle showed a bimalleolar ankle fracture that required closed manipulative reduction, intermediate suturing of the scalp and simple suturing of the arm laceration. Provide CPT codes for the procedures done in the emergency department for the facility bill.

    a. 27810, 12032

    b. 27818, 12032

    c. 27810, 12032, 12002

    d. 27810, 12032

51. The patient was admitted to the outpatient department and had a bronchoscopy with bronchial brushings performed.

    a. 31622, 31640

    b. 31622, 31623

    c. 31623

    d. 31625

52. Identify the two-digit modifier that may be reported to indicate a physician performed the postoperative management of a patient, but another physician performed the surgical procedure.

    a. –22

    b. –54

    c. –32

    d. –55

53. What is the correct CPT code assignment for destruction of internal hemorrhoids with use of infrared coagulation?

    a. 46255

    b. 46930

    c. 46260

    d. 46945

54. An encoder that takes a coder through a series of questions and choices is called a(n):

    a. Automated codebook

    b. Automated code assignment

    c. Logic-based encoder

    d. Decision support database

55. The patient was admitted with major depression severe, recurrent. What is the correct ICD-9-CM diagnosis code assignment for this condition?

    a. 296.33

    b. 296.30

    c. 311

    d. 296.89

56. A 35-year-old male was admitted with esophageal reflux. An esophagoscopy and closed esophageal biopsy was performed. Identify the code for the ICD-9-CM diagnosis and procedure.

    a. 530.89, 42.29

    b. 530.1, 45.16

    c. 530.81, 42.24

    d. 530.81, 42.23

57. Patient with flank pain was admitted and found to have a calculus of the kidney. A ureteroscopy with placement of ureteral stents was performed. Assign the correct ICD-9-CM diagnosis and procedure codes.

    a. 592.0, 788.0, 59.8

    b. 788.0, 592.0, 56.0

    c. 594.9, 59.8

    d. 592.0, 59.8

58. A female patient is admitted for stress incontinence. A urethral suspension is performed. Assign the correct ICD-9-CM diagnosis and/or procedure code(s).

    a. 625.6, 57.32

    b. 788.0, 59.5

    c. 625.6, 59.5

    d. 788.30

59. Reference codes 49491 through 49525 for inguinal hernia repair. Patient is 47 years old. What is the correct code for an initial inguinal herniorrhaphy for incarcerated hernia?

    a. 49496

    b. 49501

    c. 49507

    d. 49521

60. Patient had a laparoscopic incisional herniorrhaphy for a recurrent reducible hernia. The repair included insertion of mesh. What is the correct code assignment?

    a. 49565

    b. 49565, 49568

    c. 49656

    d. 49560, 49568

61. What is the correct CPT code assignment for hysteroscopy with lysis of intrauterine adhesions?

    a. 58555, 58559

    b. 58559

    c. 58559, 58740

    d. 58555, 58559, 58740

62. The physician performs an exploratory laparotomy with bilateral salpingo-oophorectomy. What is the correct CPT code assignment for this procedure?

    a. 49000, 58940, 58700

    b. 58940, 58720–50

    c. 49000, 58720

    d. 58720

63. Identify the CPT code for a 42-year-old diagnosed with ESRD who requires home dialysis for the month of April.

    a. 90965

    b. 90964

    c. 90966

    d. 90970

64. The patient presented to the physical therapy department and received 30 minutes of water aerobics therapeutic exercise with the therapist for treatment of arthritis. What is the appropriate treatment code(s) or modifier for a Medicare patient on a physical therapy plan of care in an outpatient setting?

    a. 97113

    b. 97113–50

    c. 97113, 97113

    d. 97110

Domain II *Reimbursement Methodologies*

65. Given the following information, which of the following statements is correct?

	MCD	Type	MS-DRG Title	Weight	Discharges	Geometric Mean	Arithmetic Mean
191	04	MED	Chronic obstructive pulmonary disease w CC	0.9757	10	4.1	5.0
192	04	MED	Chronic obstructive pulmonary disease w/o CC/MCC	0.7254	20	3.3	4.0
193	04	MED	Simple pneumonia & pleurisy w MCC	1.4327	10	5.4	6.7
194	04	MED	Simple pneumonia & pleurisy w CC	1.0056	20	4.4	5.3
195	04	MED	Simple pneumonia & pleurisy w/o CC/MCC	0.7316	10	3.5	4.1

   a. In each MS-DRG the geometric mean is lower than the arithmetic mean.

   b. In each MS-DRG the arithmetic mean is lower than the geometric mean.

   c. The higher the number of patients in each MS-DRG, the greater the geometric mean for that MS-DRG.

   d. The geometric means are lower in MS-DRGs that are associated with a CC or MCC.

66. If another status T procedure were performed, how much would the facility receive for the second status T procedure?

Billing Number	Status Indicator	CPT/HCPCS	APC
998323	V	99285–25	0612
998324	T	25500	0044
998325	X	72050	0261
998326	S	72128	0283
998327	S	70450	0283

   a. 0%

   b. 50%

   c. 75%

   d. 100%

67. A health information technician is processing payments for hospital outpatient services to be reimbursed by Medicare for a patient who had two physician visits, underwent radiology examinations, clinical laboratory tests, and who received take-home surgical dressings. Which of the following services is reimbursed under the outpatient prospective payment system?

    a. Clinical laboratory tests

    b. Physician office visits

    c. Radiology examinations

    d. Take-home surgical dressings

68. Which of the following types of hospitals are excluded from the Medicare inpatient prospective payment system?

    a. Children's

    b. Rural

    c. State supported

    d. Tertiary

69. Diagnosis-related groups are organized into:

    a. Case-mix classifications

    b. Geographic practice cost indices

    c. Major diagnostic categories

    d. Resource-based relative values

70. In processing a Medicare payment for outpatient radiology examinations, a hospital outpatient services department would receive payment under which of the following?

    a. DRGs

    b. HHRGS

    c. OASIS

    d. OPPS

71. Which of the following is *not* reimbursed according to the Medicare outpatient prospective payment system?

    a. CMHC partial hospitalization services

    b. Critical access hospitals

    c. Hospital outpatient departments

    d. Vaccines provided by CORFs

72. Fee schedules are updated by third-party payers:

    a. Annually

    b. Monthly

    c. Semiannually

    d. Weekly

73. Which of the following would a health record technician use to perform the billing function for a physician's office?

    a. CMS-1500

    b. UB-04

    c. UB-92

    d. CMS 1450

74. When a provider accepts assignment, this means the:

    a. Patient authorizes payment to be made directly to the provider

    b. The provider agrees to accept as payment in full the allowed charge from the fee schedule

    c. Balance billing is allowed on patient accounts, but at a limited rate

    d. Participating provider receives a fee-for-service reimbursement

75. A coding audit shows that an inpatient coder is using multiple codes that describe the individual components of a procedure rather than using a single code that describes all the steps of the procedure performed. Which of the following should be done in this case?

    a. Require all coders to implement this practice

    b. Report the practice to the OIG

    c. Counsel the coder and stop the practice immediately

    d. Put the coder on unpaid leave of absence

76. Prospective payment systems were developed by the federal government to:

    a. Increase healthcare access

    b. Manage Medicare and Medicaid costs

    c. Implement managed care programs

    d. Eliminate fee-for-service programs

77. Given NCCI edits, if the placement of a catheter is billed along with the performance of an infusion procedure for the same date of service for an outpatient beneficiary, Medicare will pay for:

    a. The placement of the catheter

    b. The placement of the catheter and the infusion procedure

    c. The infusion procedure

    d. Neither the placement of the catheter nor the infusion procedure

78. The goal of coding compliance programs is to prevent:

    a. Accusations of fraud and abuse

    b. Delays in claims processing

    c. Billing errors

    d. Inaccurate code assignments

79. Which of the following actions would be best to determine whether present on admission (POA) indicators for the conditions selected by CMS are having a negative impact on the hospital's Medicare reimbursement?

   a. Identify all records for a period having these indicators for these conditions and determine if these conditions are the only secondary diagnoses present on the claim that will lead to higher payment.

   b. Identify all records for a period that have these indicators for these conditions.

   c. Identify all records for a period that have these indicators for these conditions and determine whether or not additional documentation can be submitted to Medicare to increase reimbursement.

   d. Take a random sample of records for a period of time for records having these indicators for these conditions and extrapolate the negative impact on Medicare reimbursement.

80. From the information provided, how many APCs would this patient have?

Billing Number	Status Indicator	CPT/HCPCS	APC
998323	V	99285–25	0612
998324	T	25500	0044
998325	X	72050	0261
998326	S	72128	0283
998327	S	70450	0283

   a. 1

   b. 4

   c. 5

   d. 3

81. If a patient's total outpatient bill is $500, and the patient's healthcare insurance plan pays 80% of the allowable charges, what is the amount for which the patient is responsible?

   a. $10

   b. $40

   c. $100

   d. $400

82. In a managed fee-for-service arrangement, which of the following would be used as a cost-control process for inpatient surgical services?

   a. Prospectively precertify the necessity of inpatient services

   b. Determine what services can be bundled

   c. Pay only 80% of the inpatient bill

   d. Require the patient to pay 20% of the inpatient bill

83. The sum of a hospital's total relative DRG weights for a year was 15,192 and the hospital had 10,471 total discharges for the year. Given this information, what would be the hospital's case-mix index for that year?

   a. 0.689

   b. 1.59

   c. 1.45×100

   d. 1.45

84. In processing a bill under the Medicare outpatient prospective payment system (OPPS) in which a patient had three surgical procedures performed during the same operative session, which of the following would apply?

    a. Bundling of services

    b. Outlier adjustment

    c. Pass-through payment

    d. Discounting of procedures

85. A request for reconsideration of a denied claim for insurance coverage for healthcare services is called a(n):

    a. Breach

    b. Exclusion

    c. Appeal

    d. Inclusion

86. A denial of a claim is possible for all of the following reasons *except:*

    a. Not meeting medical necessity

    b. Billing too many units of a specific service

    c. Unbundling

    d. Approved precertification

87. Promoting correct coding and control of inappropriate payments is the basis of NCCI claims processing edits that help identify claims not meeting medical necessity. The NCCI automated prepayment edits used by payers is based on all of the following *except:*

    a. Coding conventions defined in the CPT book

    b. National and local policies and coding edits

    c. Analysis of standard medical and surgical practice

    d. Clinical documentation in the discharge summary

88. The NCCI editing system used in processing OPPS claims is referred to as:

    a. Outpatient code editor (OCE)

    b. Outpatient national editor (ONE)

    c. Outpatient perspective payment editor (OPPE)

    d. Outpatient claims editor (OCE)

89. Denials of outpatient claims are often generated from all of the following edits *except:*

    a. NCCI (National Correct Coding Initiative)

    b. OCE (outpatient code editor)

    c. OCE (outpatient claims editor)

    d. National and local policies

90. Timely and correct reimbursement is dependent on:

    a. Adjudication

    b. Clean claims

    c. Remittance advice

    d. Actual charge

91. Common errors that delay, rather than prevent, payment, include all of the following *except:*

    a. Patient name or certificate number

    b. Claims out of sequence

    c. Illogical demographic data

    d. Inaccurate or deleted codes

92. Which of the following is *not* an essential data element for a healthcare insurance claim?

    a. Revenue code

    b. Procedure code

    c. Provider name

    d. Procedure name

93. The next generation of consumer-directed healthcare will be driven by a design where copayments are set based on the value of the clinical services rather than the traditional practices that focus only on costs of clinical services. What new design will focus on both the benefit and cost?

    a. Value-based insurance design (VBID)

    b. Cost-based reimbursement (CBR)

    c. Pay for performance design (PPD)

    d. Prospective payment system (PPS)

94. Effective October 16, 2003, under the Administrative Simplification Compliance section of the Health Insurance Portability and Accountability Act of 1996 (HIPAA), all healthcare providers must electronically submit claims to Medicare. Which is the electronic format for hospital technical fees?

    a. 837I

    b. 837P

    c. UB-04

    d. 1500

95. What is the process that determines how a claim will be reimbursed based on the insurance benefit?

    a. Transaction

    b. Processing

    c. Adjudication

    d. Allowance

96. When clean claims are submitted, they can be adjudicated in many ways through computer software automatically. Which statement is *not* one of the outcomes that can occur as part of auto-adjudication?

    a. Auto-pay

    b. Auto-suspend

    c. Auto-calculate

    d. Auto-deny

97. What system assigns each service a value representing the true resources involved in producing it, including the time and intensity of work, the expenses of practice, and the risk of malpractice?

    a. DRGs

    b. RVUs

    c. CPT

    d. SVR

98. What statement is *not* reflective of meeting medical necessity requirements?

    a. A service or supply provided for the diagnosis, treatment, cure, or relief of a health condition, illness, injury, or disease.

    b. A service or supply provided that is not experimental, investigational, or cosmetic in purpose.

    c. A service provided that is necessary for and appropriate to the diagnosis, treatment, cure, or relief of a health condition, illness, injury, disease, or its symptoms.

    d. A service provided solely for the convenience of the insured, the insured's family, or the provider.

99. A patient has two health insurance policies: Medicare and a Medicare supplement. Which of the following statements is true?

    a. Patient receives any monies paid by the insurance companies over and above the charges.

    b. Coordination of benefits is necessary to determine which policy is primary and which is secondary so that there is no duplication of payments.

    c. The decision on which company is primary is based on remittance advice.

    d. Patient should not have a Medicare supplement.

100. What system reimburses hospitals a predetermined amount for each Medicare inpatient admission?

    a. APR-DRG

    b. DRG

    c. APC

    d. RUG

101. Medicare Part D pays for:

    a. Physician office visits

    b. Durable medical equipment

    c. Inpatient hospital care

    d. Prescription drugs

102. Medicaid is a government-sponsored healthcare insurance program that became effective in 1966 as Title 19 of the Social Security Act. Medicaid is administered by:

a. The federal government

b. The state government

c. The federal and state government

d. Third-party administrators

103. A national dollar amount that Congress designates to convert relative value units into dollars is called:

a. Conversion factor

b. Origination fee

c. Limitation factor

d. National exchange

104. The MS-DRG system creates a hospital's case-mix index (types or categories of patients treated by the hospital) based on the relative weights of the MS-DRG. The case mix can be figured by multiplying the relative weight of each MS-DRG by the number of within that MS-DRG.

a. Admissions

b. Discharges

c. CCs

d. MCCs

105. Under the Medicare hospital outpatient perspective payment system (OPPS), services are paid according to:

a. A fee-for-service schedule basis that varies according to the MPFS

b. A rate-per-service basis that varies according to the ambulatory payment classification (APC) group to which the service is assigned

c. A cost-to-charge ratio based on the hospital cost report

d. A rate-per-service basis that varies according to the DRG group

106. Under the OPPS, on which code set is the APC system primarily based for outpatient procedures and services including devices, drugs, and other covered items?

a. CPT/HCPCS

b. ICD-9-CM

c. CDT

d. MS-DRG

107. Sometimes hospital departments must work together to solve claims issue errors to prevent them from happening over and over again. What departments would need to work together if an audit found that the claim did not contain the procedure code or charge for a pacemaker insertion?

a. Health Information and Business Office

b. Health Information and Materials Management

c. Health Information, Business Office, and Cardiac Department

d. Health Information and Radiology

108. Medicare's newest claims processing payment contract entities are referred to as:

    a. Recovery audit contractors (RACs)

    b. Medicare administrative contractors (MACs)

    c. Fiscal intermediaries (FIs)

    d. Office of Inspector General contractors (OIGCs)

109. Which of the following best describes the type of coding utilized when a CPT/HCPCS code is assigned directly through the charge description master for claim submission and bypasses the record review and code assignment by the facility coding staff?

    a. Hard coding

    b. Soft coding

    c. Encoder coding

    d. Natural-language processing coding

110. What is a guarantor?

    a. The patient who is an inpatient

    b. The person responsible for the bill, such as a parent

    c. The person who bills the patient, such as the Medicare biller

    d. The patient who is an outpatient

Domain III   *Health Records and Data Content*

111. Which of the following elements is *not* a component of most patient records?

    a. Patient identification

    b. Clinical history

    c. Financial information

    d. Test results

112. Identify where the following information would be found in the acute-care record: Following induction of an adequate general anesthesia, and with the patient supine on the padded table, the left upper extremity was prepped and draped in the standard fashion.

    a. Anesthesia report

    b. Physician progress notes

    c. Operative report

    d. Recovery room record

113. Identify where the following information would be found in the acute-care record: "CBC: WBC 12.0, RBC 4.65, HGB 14.8, HCT 43.3, MCV 93."

    a. Medical laboratory report

    b. Pathology report

    c. Physical examination

    d. Physician orders

114. Identify where the following information would be found in the acute-care record: "PA and Lateral Chest: The lungs are clear. The heart and mediastinum are normal in size and configuration. There are minor degenerative changes of the lower thoracic spine."

    a. Medical laboratory report

    b. Physical examination

    c. Physician progress note

    d. Radiography report

115. The following is documented in an acute-care record: "HEENT: Reveals the tympanic membranes, nares, and pharynx to be clear. No obvious head trauma. CHEST: Good bilateral chest sounds." In which of the following would this documentation appear?

    a. History

    b. Pathology report

    c. Physical examination

    d. Operation report

116. The following is documented in an acute-care record: "Microscopic: Sections are of squamous mucosa with no atypia." In which of the following would this documentation appear?

    a. History

    b. Pathology report

    c. Physical examination

    d. Operation report

117. The following is documented in an acute-care record: "Admit to 3C. Diet: NPO. Meds: Compazine 10 mg IV Q 6 PRN." In which of the following would this documentation appear?

    a. Admission order

    b. History

    c. Physical examination

    d. Progress notes

118. The following is documented in an acute-care record: "38 weeks gestation, Apgars 8/9, 6# 9.8 oz, good cry." In which of the following would this documentation appear?

    a. Admission note

    b. Clinical laboratory

    c. Newborn record

    d. Physician order

119. The following is documented in an acute-care record: "Atrial fibrillation with rapid ventricular response, left axis deviation, left bundle branch block." In which of the following would this documentation appear?

    a. Admission order

    b. Clinical laboratory report

    c. ECG report

    d. Radiology report

120. The following is documented in an acute-care record: "I was asked to evaluate this Level I trauma patient with an open left humeral epicondylar fracture. Recommendations: Proceed with urgent surgery for debridement, irrigation, and treatment of open fracture." In which of the following would this documentation appear?

    a. Admission note

    b. Consultation report

    c. Discharge summary

    d. Nursing progress notes

121. The following is documented in an acute-care record: "Spoke to the attending re: my assessment. Provided adoption and counseling information. Spoke to CPS re: referral. Case manager to meet with patient and family." In which of the following would this documentation appear?

    a. Admission note

    b. Nursing note

    c. Physician progress note

    d. Social work note

122. Mary Smith, RHIA, has been charged with the responsibility of designing a data collection form to be used on admission of a patient to the acute-care hospital in which she works. The first resource that she should use is:

    a. UHDDS

    b. UACDS

    c. MDS

    d. ORYX

123. Both HEDIS and the Joint Commission's ORYX programs are designed to collect data to be used for:

    a. Performance-improvement programs

    b. Billing and claims data processing

    c. Developing hospital discharge abstracting systems

    d. Developing individual care plans for residents

124. A notation for a diabetic patient in a physician progress note reads: "Occasionally gets hungry. No insulin reactions. Says she is following her diabetic diet." In which part of a POMR progress note would this notation be written?

    a. Subjective

    b. Objective

    c. Assessment

    d. Plan

125. A notation for a diabetic patient in a physician progress note reads: "FBS 110 mg%, urine sugar, no acetone." In which part of a POMR progress note would this notation be written?

    a. Subjective

    b. Objective

    c. Assessment

    d. Plan

126. A notation for a hypertensive patient in a physician ambulatory care progress note reads: "Continue with Diuril, 500 mgs once daily. Return visit in 2 weeks." In which part of a POMR progress note would this notation be written?

    a. Subjective

    b. Objective

    c. Assessment

    d. Plan

127. A notation for a hypertensive patient in a physician ambulatory care progress note reads: "Blood pressure adequately controlled." In which part of a POMR progress note would this notation be written?

    a. Subjective

    b. Objective

    c. Assessment

    d. Plan

128. Reviewing the health record for missing signatures, missing medical reports, and ensuring that all documents belong in the health record is an example of _____ review.

    a. Quantitative

    b. Qualitative

    c. Statistical

    d. Outcomes

129. Dr. Jones entered a progress note in a patient's health record 24 hours after he visited the patient. Which quality element is missing from the progress note?

    a. Data completeness

    b. Data relevancy

    c. Data currency

    d. Data precision

130. The admitting data of Mrs. Smith's health record indicated that her birth date was March 21, 1948. On the discharge summary, Mrs. Smith's birth date was recorded as July 21, 1948. Which quality element is missing from Mrs. Smith's health record?

    a. Data completeness

    b. Data consistency

    c. Data accessibility

    d. Data comprehensiveness

131. Which of the following is an example of clinical data?

    a. Admitting diagnosis

    b. Date and time of admission

    c. Insurance information

    d. Health record number

132. Documentation of aides who assist a patient with activities of daily living, bathing, laundry, and cleaning would be found in which type of specialty record?

    a. Home health

    b. Behavioral health

    c. End-stage renal disease

    d. Rehabilitative care

133. Which of the following materials is *not* documented in an emergency care record?

    a. Patient's instructions at discharge

    b. Time and means of the patient's arrival

    c. Patient's complete medical history

    d. Emergency care administered before arrival at the facility

134. Which of the following provides macroscopic and microscopic information about tissue removed during an operative procedure?

    a. Anesthesia report

    b. Laboratory report

    c. Operative report

    d. Pathology report

135. What is the defining characteristic of an integrated health record format?

    a. Each section of the record is maintained by the patient care department that provided the care.

    b. Integrated health records are intended to be used in ambulatory settings.

    c. Integrated health records include both paper forms and computer printouts.

    d. Integrated health record components are arranged in strict chronological order.

136. Which of the following represents documentation of the patient's current and past health status?

    a. Physical examination

    b. Medical history

    c. Physician orders

    d. Patient consent

137. Which of the following contains the physician's findings based on an examination of the patient?

    a. Physical examination

    b. Discharge summary

    c. Medical history

    d. Patient instructions

138. What is the function of a consultation report?

    a. Provides a chronological summary of the patient's medical history and illness

    b. Documents opinions about the patient's condition from the perspective of a physician not previously involved in the patient's care

    c. Concisely summarizes the patient's treatment and stay in the hospital

    d. Documents the physician's instructions to other parties involved in providing care to a patient

139. What is the function of physician's orders?

    a. Provide a chronological summary of the patient's illness and treatment

    b. Document the patient's current and past health status

    c. Document the physician's instructions to other parties involved in providing care to a patient

    d. Document the provider's follow-up care instructions given to the patient or patient's caregiver

140. Which type of patient care record includes documentation of a family bereavement period?

    a. Hospice record

    b. Home health record

    c. Long-term care record

    d. Ambulatory care record

Domain IV *Compliance*

141. In a joint effort of the Department of Health and Human Services (DHHS), Office of Inspector General (OIG), Centers for Medicare and Medicaid Services (CMS), and Administration on Aging (AOA), which program was released in 1995 to target fraud and abuse among healthcare providers?

    a. Operation Restore Trust

    b. Medicare Integrity Program

    c. Tax Equity and Fiscal Responsibility Act (TEFRA)

    d. Medicare and Medicaid Patient and Program Protection Act

142. All of the following should be part of the core areas of a coding compliance plan *except:*

    a. Physician query process

    b. Correct use of encoder software

    c. Coding diagnoses supported by medical record documentation

    d. Tracking length of stay

143. Common forms of fraud and abuse include all of the following *except:*

    a. Upcoding

    b. Unbundling or "exploding" charges

    c. Refiling claims after denials

    d. Billing for services not furnished to patients

144. What is the primary use of the case-mix index?

    a. Benchmark of emergency room levels

    b. Defines how a hospital compares to peers and whether the facility is at risk

    c. Audit of APCS and the comparison to same-size hospitals

    d. A tool for the coding manager to compare coder productivity

145. What resource can managers use to discover current, hot areas of compliance?

   a. Policies and Procedures

   b. National Coverage Determinations

   c. Official Coding Guidelines

   d. OIG Workplan

146. This is a program unveiled in 1998 by the OIG that encourages healthcare providers to report fraudulent conduct affecting Medicare, Medicaid, and other federal healthcare programs.

   a. World Health Organization

   b. Voluntary Disclosure Program

   c. Compliance Disclosure Program

   d. Fraud and Abuse Program

147. What is the process used to transform text into an unintelligible string of characters that can be transmitted via communications media with a high degree of security and then decrypted when it reaches a secure destination?

   a. Distortion

   b. Extrication

   c. Encryption

   d. Encoded

148. Using uniform terminology is a way to improve:

   a. Validity

   b. Data timeliness

   c. Audit trails

   d. Data reliability

149. The _____ mandated the development of standards for electronic medical records.

   a. Medicare and Medicaid legislation of 1965

   b. Prospective Payment Act of 1983

   c. Health Insurance Portability and Accountability Act (HIPAA) of 1996

   d. Balanced Budget Act of 1997

150. Messaging standards for electronic data interchange in healthcare have been developed by:

   a. HL7

   b. IEE

   c. The Joint Commission

   d. CMS

151. What is the incentive to improve the quality of clinical outcomes using the electronic health record that could result in additional reimbursement or eligibility for grants or other subsidies to support further HIT efforts?

   a. Pay for performance and quality

   b. Patient referrals

   c. Payer of last resort

   d. Performance evaluations

152. A threat to data security is:

    a. Encryption

    b. Malware

    c. Audit trail

    d. Data quality

153. Data security refers to:

    a. Guaranteeing privacy

    b. Controlling access

    c. Using uniformed terminology

    d. Transparency

154. A record of all transactions in the computer system that is maintained and reviewed for unauthorized access is called a(n):

    a. Security breach

    b. Audit trail

    c. Unauthorized access

    d. Privacy trail

155. Which of the following is a true statement about data stewardship?

    a. HIM professionals are not qualified to address data stewardship issues.

    b. Data stewardship addresses the needs of the healthcare organization but not the patient.

    c. HIM professionals have worked with many data stewardship issues for years.

    d. Data stewardship does not include privacy issues.

156. A coding audit shows that an inpatient coder is using multiple codes that describe the individual components of a procedure rather than using a single code that describes all the steps of the procedure performed. Which of the following should be done in this case?

    a. Require all coders to implement this practice

    b. Report the practice to the OIG

    c. Counsel the coder and stop the practice immediately

    d. Put the coder on unpaid leave of absence

157. A health information technician (HIT) is hired as the chief compliance officer for a large group practice. In evaluating the current program, the HIT learns that there are written standards of conduct and policies and procedures that address specific areas of potential fraud as well as audits in place to monitor compliance. Which of the following should the compliance officer also ensure are in place?

    a. Compliance program education and training programs for all employees in the organization

    b. Establishment of a hotline to receive complaints and adoption of procedures to protect whistleblowers from retaliation

    c. Adopt procedures to adequately identify individuals who make complaints so that appropriate follow-up can be conducted

    d. Establish a corporate compliance committee who report directly to the CFO.

158. In developing a coding compliance program, which of the following would not be ordinarily included as participants in coding compliance education?

    a. Current coding personnel

    b. Medical staff

    c. Newly hired coding personnel

    d. Nursing staff

159. Which of the following issues compliance program guidance?

    a. AHIMA

    b. CMS

    c. Federal Register

    d. HHS Office of Inspector General (OIG)

160. The practice of assigning a diagnosis or procedure code specifically for the purpose of obtaining a higher level of payment is called:

    a. Billing

    b. Unbundling

    c. Upcoding

    d. Unnecessary service

161. This person designs, implements, and maintains a program that ensures conformity to all types of regulatory and voluntary accreditation requirements governing the provision of healthcare products or services:

    a. General Counsel

    b. Health Information Director

    c. Privacy Officer

    d. Compliance Officer

162. The HIM department is planning to scan nonelectronic medical record documentation. The project includes the scanning of health record documentation such as history and physicals, physician orders, operative reports, and nursing notes. Which of the following methods of scanning would be best to help HIM professionals monitor the completeness of health records during a patient's hospitalization?

    a. Ad hoc

    b. Concurrent

    c. Retrospective

    d. Post discharge

163. Which of the following laws created the Healthcare Integrity and Protection Data Bank?

    a. Health Information Portability and Accountability Act

    b. American Recovery and Reinvestment Act

    c. Consolidate Omnibus Budget Reconciliation Act

    d. Healthcare Quality Improvement Act

164. HIT professionals must have knowledge of:

    a. Security issues with regard to the management of healthcare reform

    b. Laws affecting the physician malpractice insurance

    c. AMA's professional ethical principles of practice regarding physician assistants

    d. Laws affecting the use of disclosure of health information

165. The HIPAA Privacy Rule:

    a. Applies to certain states

    b. Applies only to healthcare providers operated by the federal government

    c. Applies nationally to healthcare providers

    d. Serves to limit access to an individual's own health information

166. An accounting of disclosures must include disclosures:

    a. For use in law enforcement requests

    b. To any patient family member who makes a request

    c. To any individual who requested the information

    d. Made for public health reporting purposes

167. Notices of privacy practices must be available at the site where the individual is treated and:

    a. Must be posted next to the entrance

    b. Must be posted in a prominent place where it is reasonable to expect that patients will read them

    c. May be posted anywhere at the site

    d. Do not have to be posted at the site

168. Calling out patient names in a physician's office is:

    a. An incidental disclosure

    b. Not subject to the "minimum necessary" requirement

    c. A disclosure for payment purposes

    d. A HIPAA violation

Domain V *Information Technologies*

169. Which of the following is *not* an element of data quality?

    a. Accessibility

    b. Data backup

    c. Precision

    d. Relevancy

170. The protection measures and tools for safeguarding information and information systems is a definition of:

    a. Confidentiality

    b. Data security

    c. Informational privacy

    d. Informational access control

171. Computer software programs that assist in the assignment of codes used with diagnostic and procedural classifications are called:

    a. Natural-language processing systems

    b. Monitoring/audit programs

    c. Encoders

    d. Concept, description, and relationship tables

172. A special webpage that offers secure access to data is called a(n):

    a. Access control

    b. Home page

    c. Intranet

    d. Portal

173. One form of _____ uses software to aid the physician in selecting the correct code with processes such as drop-down boxes or the use of touch-screen terminals.

    a. Integrated workflow processes

    b. Computer-assisted coding

    c. Electronic document management system

    d. Speech recognition system

174. One form of _____ computer-assisted coding may use, which means that digital text from online documents stored in the information system is read directly by the software, which then suggests codes to match the documentation.

    a. Encoded vocabulary

    b. Natural-language processing

    c. Data exchange standards

    d. Structured reports

175. Which of the following tasks may *not* be performed in an electronic health record system?

    a. Document imaging

    b. Analysis

    c. Assembly

    d. Indexing

176. Electronic systems used by nurses and physicians to document assessments and findings are called:

    a. Computerized provider order entry

    b. Electronic document management systems

    c. Electronic medication administration records

    d. Electronic patient care charting

177. Data definition refers to:

    a. Meaning of data

    b. Completeness of data

    c. Consistency of data

    d. Detail of data

178. An encoder that is built using expert system techniques such as rule-based systems is a(n):

    a. Encoder interface

    b. Logic-based encoder

    c. Automated code book encoder

    d. Grouper

179. Good encoding software should include _____ to ensure data quality.

    a. Edit checks

    b. Voice recognition

    c. Reimbursement technology

    d. Passwords

180. The key data element for linking data about an individual who is seen in a variety of care settings is the:

    a. Facility medical record number

    b. Facility identification number

    c. Unique patient identifier

    d. Patient birth date

181. Which of the following make data entry easier but may harm data quality?

    a. Use of templates

    b. Copy and paste

    c. Drop-down boxes

    d. Structured data

182. A transition technology used by many hospitals to increase access to medical record content is:

    a. EHR (electronic health record)

    b. EDMS (electronic document management system)

    c. ESA (electronic signature authentication)

    d. PACS (picture archiving and communication system)

183. This system will require the author to sign onto the system using a user ID and password to complete the entries made.

    a. Digital dictation

    b. Electronic signature authentication

    c. Single sign on technology

    d. Clinical data repository

184. Coders will assign codes that have been selected into a computer program called a(n) _____ to assign the patient's case to the correct group based on ICD-9-CM and/or CPT/HCPCS codes.

    a. Encoder

    b. Computer-assisted coding

    c. Natural-language processor

    d. Grouper

Domain VI *Confidentiality and Privacy*

185. What is the legal term used to define the protection of health information in a patient–provider relationship?

    a. Access

    b. Confidentiality

    c. Privacy

    d. Security

186. The Uniform Health Care Decisions Act ranks the next-of-kin in the following order for medical decision-making purposes:

    a. Adult sibling; adult child; spouse; parent

    b. Parent; spouse; adult child; adult sibling

    c. Spouse; parent; adult sibling; adult child

    d. Spouse; adult child; parent; adult sibling

187. Which of the following is a direct command that requires an individual or a representative of an organization to appear in court or to present an object to the court?

    a. Judicial decision

    b. Subpoena

    c. Credential

    d. Regulation

188. Exceptions to the consent requirement include:

    a. Medical emergencies

    b. Provider discretion

    c. Implied consent

    d. Informed consent

189. The term *minimum necessary* means that healthcare providers and other covered entities must limit use, access, and disclosure to the minimum necessary to:

    a. Satisfy one's curiosity

    b. Accomplish the intended purpose

    c. Treat an individual

    d. Perform research

190. A well-informed patient will know that the HIPAA Privacy Rule requires that individuals be able to:

    a. Request restrictions on certain uses and disclosures of PHI

    b. Remove their record from the facility

    c. Deny provider changes to their PHI

    d. Delete portions of the record they think are incorrect

191. Written or spoken permission to proceed with care is classified as:

    a. An advanced directive

    b. Formal consent

    c. Expressed consent

    d. Implied consent

192. The number that has been proposed for use as a unique patient identification number but is controversial because of confidentiality and privacy concerns is the:

    a. Social security number

    b. Unique physician identification number

    c. Health record number

    d. National provider identifier

193. Deidentified information:

    a. Does identify an individual

    b. Is information from which personal characteristics have been stripped

    c. Can be later constituted or combined to re identify an individual

    d. Pertains to a person that is identified within the information

194. Which of the following is *not* true of notices of privacy practices?

    a. They must be made available at the site where the individual is treated.

    b. They must be posted in a prominent place.

    c. They must contain content that may not be changed.

    d. They must be prominently posted on the covered entity's website when the entity has one.

195. With regard to training in PHI policies and procedures, the following statement is true:

    a. Every member of the covered entity's workforce must be trained.

    b. Only individuals employed by the covered entity must be trained.

    c. Training only needs to occur when there are material changes to the policies and procedures.

    d. Documentation of training is not required.

196. Which document directs an individual to bring originals or copies of records to court?

    a. Summons

    b. Subpoena

    c. Subpoena duces tecum

    d. Deposition

197. To comply with HIPAA, under usual circumstances, a covered entity must act on a patient's request to review or copy his or her health information within _____ days.

    a. 10

    b. 20

    c. 30

    d. 60

198. The HIPAA Privacy Rule requires that covered entities must limit use, access, and disclosure of PHI to only the amount needed to accomplish the intended purpose. What concept is this an example of?

    a. Minimum Necessary

    b. Notice of Privacy Practices

    c. Authorization

    d. Consent

199. Which of the following statements is *false*?

    a. A notice of privacy practices must be written in plain language.

    b. Consent for use and disclosure of information must be obtained from every patient.

    c. An authorization does not have to be obtained for uses and disclosures for treatment, payment, and operations.

    d. A notice of privacy practices must give an example of a use or disclosure for healthcare operations.

200. Which of the following statements is *not* true about a business associate agreement?

    a. It prohibits the business associate from using or disclosing PHI for any purpose other than that described in the contract with the covered entity.

    b. It allows the business associate to maintain PHI indefinitely.

    c. It prohibits the business associate from using or disclosing PHI in any way that would violate the HIPAA Privacy Rule.

    d. It requires the business associate to make available all of its books and records relating to PHI use and disclosure to the Department of Health and Human Services or its agents.

CCA

PRACTICE CASE STUDIES

AMBULATORY CASE—PATIENT 1

FACE SHEET

DATE OF ADMISSION: 4/5   **DATE OF DISCHARGE:** 4/5

SEX: Male   **AGE:** 37   **DISCHARGE DISPOSITION:** Home

ADMISSION DIAGNOSIS: Left inguinal hernia

DISCHARGE DIAGNOSIS: Same

PROCEDURES: Left inguinal herniorrhaphy with excision of lipoma of spermatic cord

HISTORY AND PHYSICAL EXAMINATION—PATIENT 1

ADMITTED: 4/5

HISTORY OF PRESENT ILLNESS: The patient has been well until several months ago when he began to have pain when lifting.

PAST MEDICAL HISTORY: The patient has no other significant medical or surgical history.

SOCIAL HISTORY: Does not use alcohol or tobacco.

ALLERGIES: No known allergies

MEDICATIONS: None

REVIEW OF SYSTEMS:

    SKIN: Warm and dry, mucous membranes moist

    HEENT: Essentially normal

    LUNGS: Clear to percussion and auscultation

    HEART: Normal, regular rhythm

    ABDOMEN: Normal

    GENITALIA: Palpable mass in inguinal canal

    RECTAL: Normal

    EXTREMITIES: No edema

    NEUROLOGIC: Deep tendon reflexes normal

IMPRESSION: Left inguinal hernia

PLAN: Surgical repair of inguinal hernia

PROGRESS NOTES—PATIENT 1

DATE	NOTE
4/5	Nursing: Betadine scrub performed, patient anxious to get surgery over; preoperative medications given as ordered.
4/5	Attending MD: Brief op note Dx: Left inguinal hernia Px: Left inguinal herniorrhaphy Anes: Local plus sedation Complications: None
4/5	Attending MD: No bleeding; patient okay for discharge.

OPERATIVE REPORT—PATIENT 1

DATE: 4/5

PREOPERATIVE DIAGNOSIS: Left direct inguinal hernia

POSTOPERATIVE DIAGNOSIS: Left direct inguinal hernia

OPERATION: Left inguinal herniorrhaphy

ANESTHESIA: Local plus sedation

OPERATIVE INDICATIONS: A wide mouth direct sac was present in the lower inguinal canal. A lipoma of the cord was present, but no indirect sac.

OPERATIVE PROCEDURE: Under local anesthesia consisting of the equivalent of 19 cc of 1% Xylocaine and 8 cc of 0.5% Marcaine, the abdomen was prepared with Betadine and sterilely draped. A left inguinal incision was made and carried down through subcutaneous tissues to the aponeurosis of the external oblique, which was opened from the external ring to a point over the internal ring. Flaps were cleaned in both directions. The nerve was retracted inferiorly. The cord structures were separated from the surrounding at the level of the pubic tubercle and retracted with a Penrose drain. Cremaster over the cord was opened and a search made for an indirect sac. None was found. Lipoma of the cord was dissected free and clamped at its base and excised. The base was ligated with 00 chromic catgut. Additional cremasteric muscles were divided and ligated with 00 chromic catgut. The direct sac was further dissected down to its base and inverted as the defect was closed by approximating transversus to transversus with a running suture of 00 Vicryl. The floor of the canal was then closed by approximating the internal oblique to the shelving portion of the inguinal ligament with multiple sutures of 0 Ethibond. The external oblique aponeurosis was then reclosed with 0 Ethibond, leaving the cord and nerve in the subcutaneous position. Several sutures of 0 Ethibond were also placed above the emergence of the cord at the internal ring. Subcutaneous tissues were then approximated with 3-0 Vicryl and after irrigation skin was closed with skin clips. The patient tolerated the procedure well and was sent to the recovery room in good condition.

PATHOLOGY REPORT—PATIENT 1

DATE SPECIMEN SUBMITTED: 4/5

SPECIMEN: Lipoma of cord

CLINICAL DATA:

GROSS DESCRIPTION: The specimen is submitted as lipoma of cord. It consists of a single irregularly shaped fragment of fatty tissue that is $8.0 \times 4.0 \times 1.5$ cm. It is covered with a thin membrane.

MICROSCOPIC DESCRIPTION:

DIAGNOSIS: Lipomatous tissue of left spermatic cord

PHYSICIAN'S ORDERS—PATIENT 1

DATE	ORDER
4/5	Attending MD:
	Admit to same-day surgery
	Betadine scrub ×3 Preop
	May take own meds
4/5	Anesthesia note:
	Continue NPO
	Demerol 50 mg IM 1½ hr Preop
	Vistaril 50 mg IM 1½ hr Preop
	Atropine 0.4 mg IM 1½ hr Preop
4/5	Attending MD:
	Vital signs q. 15 min until stable
	Regular diet
	Darvocet-N-100 q. 4 hrs p.r.n. pain
	Discharge to home when stable

LABORATORY REPORTS—PATIENT 1

HEMATOLOGY

DATE: 4/5

Specimen	Results	Normal Values
WBC	6.83	4.3–11.0
RBC	4.57	4.5–5.9
HGB	13.7	13.5–17.5
HCT	43	41–52
MCV	87.0	80–100
MCHC	35	31–57
PLT	300	150–400

AUTO DIFFERENTIAL—PATIENT 1

DATE: 4/5

Specimen	Results	Normal Values
NEUT	68.3	40.0–74.0
LYMPH	20	19.0–48.0
MONO	5.6	3.4–9.0
EOS	5.6	0.0–7.0
BASO	0.6	0.0–1.5
LUC	3.8	0.0–4.0

URINALYSIS—PATIENT 1

DATE: 4/5

Test	Result	Ref Range
SP GRAVITY	1.017	1.005–1.035
PH	6	5–7
PROT	TRACE	NEG
GLUC	NONE	NEG
KETONES	NONE	NEG
BILI	NONE	NEG
BLOOD	TRACE	NEG
NITRATES	NONE	NEG
RBCS	NONE	NEG
WBCS	NONE	NEG

RADIOLOGY REPORT—PATIENT 1

DATE: 4/5

DIAGNOSIS: Inguinal hernia

EXAMINATION: Chest x-ray

Heart size and shape are acceptable. The lung fields are clear and the pulmonary vascular pattern is unremarkable. There is no free fluid and the trachea remains midline.

Enter two diagnosis codes and two procedure codes.

PDX

DX2

PP1

PR2

AMBULATORY RECORD—PATIENT 2

DATE: 8/12/20XX

SURGERY RECORD:

PATIENT HISTORY: This patient is seen today to insert an intrathecal pump for pain management due to ductal carcinoma of the left upper breast metastatic to the spine. She previously underwent modified radical mastectomy with general anesthesia and had no adverse effects. No other surgical history is given. No known allergies, no current medications. Review of systems is normal ASA = 2.

Following preoperative evaluation and discussion with the patient, local anesthesia was used to implant an intrathecal programmable pump surgically placed and attached to a previously placed catheter. The patient tolerated the procedure well. There were no adverse effects of anesthesia.

Enter three diagnosis codes and one procedure code.

PDX

DX2

DX3

PP1

AMBULATORY RECORD—PATIENT 3

PREOPERATIVE DIAGNOSIS: Reflex sympathetic dystrophy, left knee

POSTOPERATIVE DIAGNOSIS: Reflex sympathetic dystrophy, left knee

OPERATION: Left lumbar sympathetic block with C-arm

ANESTHESIA: Local

INDICATIONS:

This 43-year-old female has a 7-month history of left knee pain. She says that even a light touch appears to be exquisitely painful. She has had surgery to clear scar tissue.

PROCEDURE DESCRIPTION:

The patient was placed on the x-ray lucent gurney in the right lateral decubitus position. The back was prepped with Betadine, and the midline spinous processes were marked. A line was drawn 6 to 7 cm lateral to that midline on the left. L2 was identified using the C-arm and lateral projections, and lidocaine was infiltrated at the skin. The 22-gauge, 6-inch Chiba needle was advanced down to and off the body of L2, and loss of resistance was obtained with a glass syringe. Renografin-60 was injected and showed a good distribution. So 15 cc of bupivacaine 0.5% without epinephrine was injected, plus Depo-Medrol 40 mg. The needle was withdrawn.

Then lidocaine was infiltrated on the 6- to 7-cm line at L4. I advanced the 22-gauge, 6-inch needle off the body of L4, but the Renografin-60 distribution appeared not to be adequate. Another wheal was raised at the 13 level, and the needle was advanced down to and off the body of L3. A loss of resistance was obtained with a glass syringe, followed by Renografin-60. This time, the distribution was excellent, and bupivacaine 0.5% without epinephrine =15 cc was injected. She was left on her side for 25 minutes. After 10 minutes, she had a noticeably warmer left foot and ankle. The skin coloration of the left leg was normal.

Enter one diagnosis code and two procedure codes.

PDX

PP1

PR2

INPATIENT RECORD—PATIENT 4

DISCHARGE SUMMARY

DATE OF ADMISSION: 9/8   **DATE OF DISCHARGE:** 9/10

DISCHARGE DIAGNOSIS:

1. Acute pyelonephritis

2. Septicemia, resistant to ampicillin and penicillin

ADMISSION HISTORY: This 21-year-old female was admitted to the hospital with discomfort in the right side. Other than this she has been healthy. On the day of admission she developed severe discomfort in the lower back. She was having fever and chills for which she took an aspirin and then she came to the emergency department.

COURSE IN HOSPITAL: The patient was treated with intravenous antibiotics in the form of gentamicin and cefoxitin. She continued to improve on this regimen and became afebrile after about three days of treatment. Her physical examination remained essentially unchanged; however, there was marked improvement in the patient's general condition. The patient also had an onset of herpes simplex infection on her upper lip, for which she was given Zovirax ointment.

INSTRUCTIONS ON DISCHARGE: The patient was discharged home on ciprofloxacin 500 mg p.o. b.i.d. × 12 days. A repeat blood culture done just prior to discharge showed no growth at the end of 7 days. She is to be followed up in my office in about a week after discharge to have a repeat urine culture done. The patient was also given a prescription for Zyban to assist smoking cessation.

HISTORY AND PHYSICAL EXAMINATION—PATIENT 4

ADMITTED: 9/8

REASON FOR ADMISSION: This was the first hospital admission for this 21-year-old white female, who experienced difficulty about 3 days prior to admission. This was in the form of discomfort in the right side of the lower back and also some dysuria. On the evening of admission, she started experiencing some fever and chills and took some aspirin. This did not help her and she came to the emergency department.

HISTORY OF PRESENT ILLNESS:

PAST MEDICAL HISTORY: Remarkable only for "walking pneumonia" treated with erythromycin 3 months ago. She also suffered contusion of her right kidney after a fall from a horse about 4 years prior to admission.

ALLERGIES: None known

CHRONIC MEDICATIONS: None

FAMILY HISTORY: Remarkable for multiple members of the family having seasonal allergies

SOCIAL HISTORY: The patient lives with two friends and is employed by a saddle shop. She drinks about one drink a week and smokes a pack of cigarettes a day.

REVIEW OF SYSTEMS: The patient relates that there has been no weight gain or loss and that she was well functioning until three days ago when she developed lower back pain, primarily on the right side. She also relates that she has had dysuria for this same time period.

HISTORY AND PHYSICAL EXAMINATION—PATIENT 4 (continued)

PHYSICAL EXAMINATION: On admission, significant for temperature of 103 degrees; pulse 120 beats per minute, regular; blood pressure 120/70; respirations 16

VITAL SIGNS: P 120/min, regular; BP 120/70; Temp 103 degrees; R 16/min, regular

GENERAL: The patient is a well-developed female of her stated age. She appears lethargic but responsive. The patient appears septic.

SKIN: Warm to touch

HEENT: Pupils equal, react briskly to light. Mucous membranes of the eyes, nose, mouth, and oropharynx are normal.

NECK: Supple, trachea is central, the carotid pulses are symmetrical. There is no goiter.

LUNGS: Clear to auscultation and percussion

BACK: Positive pain to palpation and percussion right costovertebral angle

HEART: Peripheral pulses are symmetrical. The cardiac apex is not displaced. The heart sounds are normal and there are no added sounds or murmurs.

ABDOMEN: Soft, nontender, with no masses palpable. The bowel sounds are normal.

GENITALIA: Normal female

RECTAL: Deferred

EXTREMITIES: Femoral pulses normal, no edema

NEUROLOGIC: Grossly intact

LABORATORY DATA: WBC 15.9 with differential of 57 Segs; 33 Bands; 6 Lymphs; 4 Monos. Electrolytes were normal. BUN 11. Urine culture grew out *E. coli*, more than 100,000 colonies per mL. Blood culture was also positive for *E. coli*. This was sensitive to gentamicin and cefoxitin, as well as many other antibiotics. Urinalysis on admission revealed many WBCs and marked bacteriuria. Chest x-ray was unremarkable.

IMPRESSION: Admit for clinical features of acute pyelonephritis and septicemia.

PLAN: Hydrate and start IV antibiotics.

PROGRESS NOTES—PATIENT 4

DATE	NOTE
9/8	Patient admitted for evaluation of flank pain and fever. She also has a lesion on her lip. This appears to be herpes simplex. Will treat infection process with antibiotics following obtaining cultures. The patient's renal function will be monitored.
9/10	The patient's fever decreasing. Patient comfortable and tolerating antibiotics. Will continue IVs. The importance of stopping cigarette use was discussed with the patient. She is willing to quit and she will be given a prescription for Zyban at discharge.
9/11	Patient is afebrile today. Will discharge when able to obtain transportation.

PHYSICIAN'S ORDERS—PATIENT 4

DATE	ORDER
9/8	Admit to floor for evaluation of febrile illness
	Urinalysis
	CBC and SMA 16
	Urine culture and sensitivity
	Blood cultures ×2
	Chest x-ray
	Pyelogram
	D5W 125 cc/h ×3
	Strict input and output
	Zovirax ointment prn to lip
	Gentamicin 80 mg IV q. 8 H ×3d
	Cefoxitin 1 g IV q. 8 H ×3 days
9/9	D5W 100 cc/ph
9/10	Discharge patient when transportation is arranged
	Ciprofloxacin 500 mg p.o. b.i.d. ×12 days
	Zyban 150 mg p.o. daily ×3 days then b.i.d.
	Follow up in the office in 1 week.

LABORATORY REPORTS—PATIENT 4

HEMATOLOGY

DATE: 9/8

Specimen	Results	Normal Values
WBC	15.9 H	4.3–11.0
RBC	5.5	4.5–5.9
HGB	14.0	13.5–17.5
HCT	45	41–52
MCV	90	80–100
MCHC	41	31–57
PLT	251	150–450

LABORATORY REPORTS—PATIENT 4 (continued)

CHEMISTRY—PATIENT 4

DATE: 9/8

Specimen	Results	Normal Values
GLUC	100	70–110
BUN	11	8–25
CREAT	1.0	0.5–1.5
NA	143	136–146
K	4.0	3.5–5.5
CL	98	95–110
CO$_2$	30	24–32
CA	9.0	8.4–10.5
PHOS	3.0	2.5–4.4
MG	2.0	1.6–3.0
T BILI	1.0	0.2–1.2
D BILI	0.3	0.0–0.5
PROTEIN	7.0	6.0–8.0
ALBUMIN	5.2	5.0–5.5
AST	25	0–40
ALT	40	30–65
GGT	60	15–85
LD		100–190
ALK PHOS		50–136
URIC ACID		2.2–7.7
CHOL		0–200
TRIG		10–160

URINALYSIS—PATIENT 4

DATE: 9/8

Test	Result	Ref Range
SP GRAVITY	1.03	1.005–1.035
PH	6	5–7
PROT	NEG	NEG
GLUC	NEG	NEG
KETONES	NEG	NEG
BILI	NEG	NEG
BLOOD	NEG	NEG
LEU EST	POS	NEG
NITRATES	POS	NEG
RED SUBS	NEG	NEG

MICROBIOLOGY—PATIENT 4

DATE	TEST TYPE: Culture and Sensitivity
9/8	SOURCE: Urine
	SITE:
	GRAM STAIN RESULTS
	CULTURE RESULTS: *E. coli*, 100,000/ml
	SUSCEPTIBILITY:

9/10		
	AMPICILLIN	R
	CEFAZOLIN	S
	CEFOTAXIME	S
	CEFTRIAXONE	S
	CEFUROXIME	S
	CEPHALOTHIN	S
	CIPROFLOXACIN	S
	ERYTHROMYCIN	S
	GENTAMICIN	S
	OXACILLIN	S
	PENICILLIN	R
	PIPERACILLIN	
	TETRACYCLINE	
	TOBRAMYCIN	
	TRIMETH/SULF	
	VANCOMYCIN	

S = SUSCEPTIBLE

R = RESISTANT

I = INTERMEDIATE

M = MODERATELY SUSCEP

LABORATORY RESULTS—PATIENT 4

DATE: 9/11

URINE CULTURE: No growth for 24 hours

MICROBIOLOGY—PATIENT 4

DATE	TEST TYPE:	
9/8	Culture and Sensitivity #1	
	SOURCE: Blood	
	SITE:	
	GRAM STAIN RESULTS	
	CULTURE RESULTS: *E. coli*	
	SUSCEPTIBILITY:	
9/10	AMPICILLIN	R
	CEFAZOLIN	S
	CEFOTAXIME	S
	CEFTRIAXONE	S
	CEFUROXIME	S
	CEPHALOTHIN	S
	CIPROFLOXACIN	S
	ERYTHROMYCIN	S
	GENTAMICIN	S
	OXACILLIN	S
	PENICILLIN	R
	PIPERACILLIN	
	TETRACYCLINE	
	TOBRAMYCIN	
	TRIMETH/SULF	
	VANCOMYCIN	

S = SUSCEPTIBLE

R= RESISTANT

I = INTERMEDIATE

M = MODERATELY SUSCEP

MICROBIOLOGY—PATIENT 4

DATE	TEST TYPE:
9/8	Culture and Sensitivity #2
	SOURCE: Blood
	SITE:
	GRAM STAIN RESULTS
	CULTURE RESULTS: *E. coli*
	SUSCEPTIBILITY:

9/10		
	AMPICILLIN	R
	CEFAZOLIN	S
	CEFOTAXIME	S
	CEFTRIAXONE	S
	CEFUROXIME	S
	CEPHALOTHIN	S
	CIPROFLOXACIN	S
	ERYTHROMYCIN	S
	GENTAMICIN	S
	OXACILLIN	S
	PENICILLIN	R
	PIPERACILLIN	
	TETRACYCLINE	
	TOBRAMYCIN	
	TRIMETH/SULF	
	VANCOMYCIN	

S = SUSCEPTIBLE

R = RESISTANT

I = INTERMEDIATE

M = MODERATELY SUSCEP

RADIOLOGY REPORT—PATIENT 4

DATE: 9/8

CHEST X-RAY: The examination is of a recumbent AP view. Heart size is normal. The aorta is normal and lung fields are free of infiltration. There is no free air and the trachea is midline.

DIAGNOSIS: Normal chest x-ray

RADIOLOGY REPORT—PATIENT 4

DATE: 9/8

PYELOGRAM: The urinary architecture is normal with no hydronephrosis.

DIAGNOSIS: Normal pyelogram

Enter five diagnosis codes.

PDX

DX2

DX3

DX4

DX5

INPATIENT RECORD—PATIENT 5

DISCHARGE SUMMARY

DATE OF ADMISSION: 2/3   **DATE OF DISCHARGE:** 2/5

DISCHARGE DIAGNOSIS: Full-term pregnancy—delivered male infant

Patient started labor spontaneously three days before her due date. She was brought to the hospital by automobile. Labor progressed for a while but then contractions became fewer and she delivered soon after. A midline episiotomy was done. Membranes and placenta were complete. There was some bleeding but not excessive. Patient made an uneventful recovery.

HISTORY AND PHYSICAL EXAMINATION—PATIENT 5

ADMITTED: 2/3

REASON FOR ADMISSION: Full-term pregnancy

PAST MEDICAL HISTORY: Previous deliveries normal and mitral valve prolapse

ALLERGIES: None known

CHRONIC MEDICATIONS: None

FAMILY HISTORY: Heart disease—father

SOCIAL HISTORY: The patient is married and has one other child living with her.

REVIEW OF SYSTEMS:

> **SKIN:** Normal
>
> **HEAD-SCALP:** Normal
>
> **EYES:** Normal
>
> **ENT:** Normal
>
> **NECK:** Normal
>
> **BREASTS:** Normal
>
> **THORAX:** Normal
>
> **LUNGS:** Normal
>
> **HEART:** Slight midsystolic click with late systolic murmur II/VI
>
> **ABDOMEN:** Normal

IMPRESSION: Good health with term pregnancy. History of mitral valve prolapse—asymptomatic.

PROGRESS NOTES—PATIENT 5

DATE	NOTE
2/3	Admit to Labor and Delivery. MVP stable. Patient progressing well.
	Delivered at 1:15 p.m. one full-term male infant.
2/4	Patient doing well. Mitral valve prolapse stable. The perineum is clean and dry, incision intact.
2/5	Will discharge to home

PHYSICIAN'S ORDERS—PATIENT 5

DATE	ORDER
2/3	Admit to Labor and Delivery
	1,000 cc 5% D/LR
	May ambulate
	Type and screen
	CBC
	May have ice chips
2/5	Discharge patient to home

DELIVERY RECORD—PATIENT 5

DATE: 2/3

The patient was 3 cm dilated when admitted. The duration of the first stage of labor was 6 hours, second stage was 14 minutes, third stage was 5 minutes. She was given local anesthesia. An episiotomy was performed with repair. There were no lacerations. The cord was wrapped once around the baby's neck, but did not cause compression. The mother and liveborn baby were discharged from the delivery room in good condition.

LABORATORY REPORT—PATIENT 5

HEMATOLOGY

DATE: 2/3

Specimen	Results	Normal Values
WBC	5.2	4.3–11.0
RBC	4.9	4.5–5.9
HGB	13.8	13.5–17.5
HCT	45	41–52
MCV	93	80–100
MCHC	41	31–57
PLT	255	150–450

Enter four diagnosis codes and one procedure code.

PDX

DX2

DX3

DX4

PP1

EMERGENCY DEPARTMENT RECORD—PATIENT 6

DATE OF ADMISSION: 8/19   DATE OF DISCHARGE: 8/19

HISTORY (Problem Focused):

ADMISSION HISTORY: This is a 13-year-old African-American male. He became short of breath, used his inhaler as described but continued to have wheezing and shortness of breath.

ALLERGIES: None

CHRONIC MEDICATIONS: Albuterol inhaler

FAMILY HISTORY: Noncontributory

SOCIAL HISTORY: The patient's father smokes one pack of cigarettes per day, but he does not smoke in the house.

REVIEW OF SYSTEMS: His integumentary, musculoskeletal, cardiovascular, genitourinary, and gastrointestinal systems are negative.

PHYSICAL EXAMINATION (Extended Problem Focused):

GENERAL APPEARANCE: This is an alert, cooperative young male in acute distress.

HEENT: PERRLA, extraocular movements are full

NECK: Supple

CHEST: Lungs reveal wheezes and rales. Heart has normal sinus rhythm.

ABDOMEN: Soft and nontender, no organomegaly

EXTREMITIES: Examination is normal.

LABORATORY DATA: Urinalysis is normal, EKG normal, chest x-ray is normal. CBC and diff show no abnormalities.

IMPRESSION: Acute asthma with exacerbation

PLAN: Administer epinephrine and intravenous theophylline

TREATMENT: Following administration of epinephrine and theophylline, the patient's asthma abated. One venipuncture set and one IV set were used to administer the medication over 30 minutes.

DISCHARGE DIAGNOSIS: Asthma with exacerbation

DISCHARGE INSTRUCTIONS: The patient was instructed to take his prescribed medications as directed by his primary care physician and to return to the ER if he had any further asthma.

Enter one diagnosis code and two procedure codes.

PDX

PP1

PR2

EXAM 1

Domain I *Clinical Classification Systems*

1. Identify the code for a patient with a closed transcervical fracture of the epiphysis.

   a. 820.09

   b. 820.02

   c. 820.03

   d. 820.01

2. Identify the ICD-9-CM diagnosis code(s) for neonatal tooth eruption.

   a. 525.0

   b. 520.6, 525.0

   c. 520.9

   d. 520.6

3. Identify CPT code(s) for the following patient. A 35-year-old female undergoes an excision of a 3.0-cm tumor in her forehead. An incision is made through the skin and subcutaneous tissue. The tumor is dissected free of surrounding structures. The wound is closed in layers with interrupted sutures.

   a. 21012

   b. 21012, 12052

   c. 21014

   d. 21014, 12052

4. Identify CPT code(s) for the following Medicare patient. A 67-year-old female undergoes a fine-needle aspiration of the left breast with ultrasound guidance to place a localization clip during a breast biopsy.

   a. 10022

   b. 10022, 19295–LT

   c. 10022, 19295–LT, 76942

   d. 10022, 76942

5. Identify the appropriate ICD-9-CM diagnosis code for Lou Gehrig's disease.

   a. 335.20

   b. 334.8

   c. 335.29

   d. 335.2

6. Identify the ICD-9-CM procedure code(s) for insertion of dual chamber cardiac pacemaker and atrial and ventricular leads.

   a. 37,83, 37.73

   b. 37.83, 37.71

   c. 37.81, 37.73, 37.71

   d. 37.83, 37.72

7. Identify the correct ICD-9-CM procedure code(s) for replacement of an old dual pacemaker with a new dual pacemaker.

   a. 37.87

   b. 37.85

   c. 37.87, 37.89

   d. 37.85, 37.89

8. Identify the appropriate ICD-9-CM diagnosis code(s) for right and left bundle branch block.

   a. 426.3, 426.4

   b. 426.53

   c. 426.4, 426.53

   d. 426.52

9. Identify the appropriate diagnostic and procedure ICD-9-CM code(s) for reprogramming of a cardiac pacemaker.

   a. V53.31

   b. 37.85

   c. V53.02

   d. V53.31, 37.85

10. This is a condition with an imprecise diagnosis with various characteristics. The condition may be diagnosed when a patient presents with sinus arrest, sinoatrial exit block, or persistent sinus bradycardia. This syndrome is often the result of drug therapy, such as digitalis, calcium channel blockers, beta-blockers, sympatholytic agents, or antiarrhythmics. Another presentation includes recurrent supraventricular tachycardias associated with bradyarrhythmias. Prolonged ambulatory monitoring may be indicated to establish a diagnosis of this condition. Treatment includes insertion of a permanent cardiac pacemaker.

    a. Atrial fibrillation (427.31)

    b. Atrial flutter (427.32)

    c. Paroxysmal supraventricular tachycardia (427.0)

    d. Sick sinus syndrome (SSS) (427.81)

11. Identify the appropriate ICD-9-CM procedure code(s) for a double internal mammary-coronary artery bypass.

    a. 36.15, 36.16

    b. 36.15

    c. 36.16

    d. 36.12, 36.16

12. Coronary arteriography serves as a diagnostic tool in detecting obstruction within the coronary arteries. Identify the technique using two catheters inserted percutaneously through the femoral artery.

    a. Combined right and left (88.54)

    b. Stones (88.55)

    c. Judkins (88.56)

    d. Other and unspecified (88.57)

13. Identify the correct diagnosis ICD-9-CM code(s) for a patient who arrives at the hospital for outpatient laboratory services ordered by the physician to monitor the patient's Coumadin levels. A prothrombin time (PT) is performed to check the patient's long-term use of his anticoagulant treatment.

    a. V58.83, V58.61

    b. V58.83, V58.63

    c. V58.61, 790.92

    d. V58.61

14. Identify the CPT code(s) for the following patient: A 2-year-old boy presented to the emergency room in the middle of the night to have his nasogastric feeding tube repositioned through the duodenum under fluoroscopic guidance.

    a. 43752

    b. 43761

    c. 43761, 76000

    d. 49450

15. Identify the CPT code(s) for the following patient: A 2-year-old boy presented to the hospital to have his gastrostomy tube changed under fluoroscopic guidance.

    a. 43752

    b. 43760

    c. 43761, 76000

    d. 49450

16. Identify the ICD-9-CM diagnosis code for blighted ovum.

    a. 236.1

    b. 661.00

    c. 631.8

    d. 634.90

17. Identify the ICD-9-CM diagnostic code(s) for the following: threatened abortion with hemorrhage at 15 weeks; home undelivered.

    a. 640.01, 640.91

    b. 640.03

    c. 640.83

    d. 640.80

32. Which of the following is (are) the correct ICD-9-CM procedure code(s) for cystoscopy with biopsy?

    a. 57.34

    b. 57.32, 57.33

    c. 57.33

    d. 57.39

Domain II *Reimbursement Methodologies*

33. Which of the following software applications would be used to aid in the coding function in a physician's office?

    a. Grouper

    b. Encoder

    c. Pricer

    d. Diagnosis calculator

34. Which payment system was introduced in 1992 and replaced Medicare's customary, prevailing, and reasonable (CPR) payment system?

    a. Diagnosis-related groups

    b. Resource-based relative value scale system

    c. Long-term care drugs

    d. Resource utilization groups

35. The patient had a total abdominal hysterectomy with bilateral salpingo-oophorectomy. The coder assigned the following codes:

    > 58150, Total abdominal hysterectomy, with/without removal of tubes and ovaries
    > 58700, Salpingectomy, complete or partial, unilateral/bilateral (separate procedure)

    What error has the coder made by using these codes?

    a. Maximizing

    b. Upcoding

    c. Unbundling

    d. Optimizing

36. What is the best reference tool to determine how CPT codes should be assigned?

    a. Local coverage determination from Medicare

    b. American Medical Association's *CPT Assistant* newsletter

    c. American Hospital Association's *Coding Clinic*

    d. CMS website

37. An electrolyte panel (80051) in the laboratory section of CPT consists of tests for carbon dioxide (82374), chloride (82435), potassium (84132), and sodium (84295). If each of the component codes are reported and billed individually on a claim form, this would be a form of:

   a. Optimizing

   b. Unbundling

   c. Sequencing

   d. Classifying

38. In the laboratory section of CPT, if a group of tests overlaps two or more panels, report the panel that incorporates the greatest number of tests to fulfill the code definition. What would a coder do with the remaining test codes that are not part of a panel?

   a. Report the remaining tests using individual test codes, according to CPT.

   b. Do not report the remaining individual test codes.

   c. Report only those test codes that are part of a panel.

   d. Do not report a test code more than once regardless whether the test was performed twice.

39. There are several codes to describe a colonoscopy. CPT code 45378 describes the most basic colonoscopy without additional services. Additional codes in the colonoscopy section of CPT further define removal of foreign body (45379); biopsy, single or multiple (45380); and others. Reporting the basic form of a colonoscopy (45378) with a foreign body (45379) or biopsy code (45380) would violate which rule?

   a. Unbundling

   b. Optimizing

   c. Sequencing

   d. Maximizing

40. What did the Centers of Medicare and Medicaid Services develop to promote national correct coding methodologies and to control improper coding leading to inappropriate payment in Part B claims?

   a. Outpatient Perspective Payment System (OPPS)

   b. National Correct Coding Initiative (NCCI)

   c. Ambulatory Payment Classifications (APCs)

   d. Comprehensive Outpatient Rehab Facilities (CORFs)

41. What is the best reference tool for ICD-9-CM coding advice?

   a. AMA's *CPT Assistant*

   b. AHA's *Coding Clinic for HCPCS*

   c. AHA's *Coding Clinic for ICD-9-CM*

   d. National Correct Coding Initiative (NCCI)

42. CMS developed medically unlikely edits (MUEs) to prevent providers from billing units of services greater than the norm would indicate. These MUEs were implemented on January 1, 2007, and are applied to which code set?

    a. Diagnosis-related groups

    b. HCPCS/CPT codes

    c. ICD-9-CM diagnosis and procedure codes

    d. Resource utilization groups

43. Several key principles require appropriate physician documentation to secure payment from the insurer. Which answer (listed here) fails to impact payment based on physician responsibility?

    a. The health record should be complete and legible.

    b. The rationale for ordering diagnostic and other ancillary services should be documented or easily inferred.

    c. Documenting the charges and services on the itemized bill.

    d. The patient's progress and response to treatment and any revision in the treatment plan and diagnoses should be documented.

44. The documentation of each patient encounter should include the following to secure payment from the insurer *except:*

    a. The reason for the encounter and the patient's relevant history, physical examination, and prior diagnostic test results

    b. A patient assessment, clinical impression, or diagnosis

    c. A plan of care

    d. The identity of the patient's nearest relative and emergency contact number

45. Two patients were hospitalized with bacterial pneumonia. One patient was hospitalized for three days, and the other patient was hospitalized for 30 days. Both cases result in the same DRG with different lengths of stay. Which answer most closely describes how the hospital will be reimbursed?

    a. The hospital will receive the same DRG for both patients but additional reimbursement will be allowed for the patient who stayed 30 days because the length of stay was greater than the geometric length of stay for this DRG.

    b. The hospital will receive the same reimbursement for the same DRG regardless of the length of stay.

    c. The hospital can appeal the payment for the patient who was in the hospital for 30 days because the cost of care was significantly higher than the average length of stay for the DRG payment.

    d. The hospital will receive a day outlier for the patient who was hospitalized for 30 days.

46. Which of the following statements are true?

    a. The higher the relative weight, the higher the payment rates.

    b. The lower the relative weight, the higher the payment rates.

    c. The lower the relative weight, the sicker the patient.

    d. The higher the relative weight, the lesser reimbursement due the facility.

47. Which classification system is in place to reimburse home health agencies?

    a. MS-DRGs

    b. RUGs

    c. HHRGs

    d. APCs

48. What reimbursement system uses the Medicare fee schedule?

    a. APCs

    b. MS-DRGs

    c. RBRVS

    d. RUG-III

49. MS diagnostic-related groups are organized into:

    a. Case-mix classifications

    b. Geographic practice cost indices

    c. Major diagnostic categories

    d. Resource-based relative values

50. Which of the following hospitals are excluded from the Medicare acute-care prospective payment system?

    a. Children's

    b. Small community

    c. Tertiary

    d. Trauma

51. CMS identified conditions that are not present on admission and could be "reasonably preventable," and therefore hospitals are not allowed to receive additional payment for these conditions that do present. What are these conditions called?

    a Conditions of Participation

    b. Present on admission

    c. Hospital-acquired conditions

    d. Hospital-acquired infection

52. Which of the following fails to meet the CMS classification of a hospital-acquired condition?

    a. Foreign object retained after surgery

    b. Air embolism

    c. Gram-negative pneumonia

    d. Blood incompatibility

53. Which of the following fails to meet the CMS classification of a hospital-acquired condition?

    a. Stage I pressure ulcers

    b. Falls and trauma

    c. Catheter-associated infection

    d. Vascular catheter–associated infection

54. The electronic claim format (837I) replaces which paper billing form?

    a. CMS-1500

    b. CMS-1450 (UB-04)

    c. UB-92

    d. CMS-1400

55. This is a statement sent by third-party payers to the patient to explain services provided, amounts billed, and payments made by the health plan.

    a. Coordination of benefits (COB)

    b. Explanation of benefits (EOB)

    c. Medicare summary notice (MSN)

    d. Remittance advice (RA)

Domain III   *Health Records and Data Content*

56. An outpatient clinic is reviewing the functionality of a computer system it is considering purchasing. Which of the following datasets should the clinic consult to ensure all the federally required data elements for Medicare and Medicaid outpatient clinical encounters are collected by the system?

    a. DEEDS

    b. EMEDS

    c. UACDS

    d. UHDDS

57. Standardizing medical terminology to avoid differences in naming various medical conditions and procedures (such as the synonyms bunionectomy, McBride procedure, and repair of hallus valgus) is one purpose of:

    a. Transaction standards

    b. Content and structure standards

    c. Vocabulary standards

    d. Security standards

58. A family practitioner requests the opinion of a physician specialist in endocrinology who reviews the patient's health record and examines the patient. The physician specialist records findings, impressions, and recommendations in which type of report?

    a. Consultation

    b. Medical history

    c. Physical examination

    d. Progress notes

59. Which of the following is *not* a function of the discharge summary?

    a. Providing information about the patient's insurance coverage

    b. Ensuring the continuity of future care

    c. Providing information to support the activities of the medical staff review committee

    d. Providing concise information that can be used to answer information requests

60. Ensuring the continuity of future care by providing information to the patient's attending physician, referring physician, and any consulting physicians is a function of the:

    a. Discharge summary

    b. Autopsy report

    c. Incident report

    d. Consent to treatment

61. A 65-year-old white male was admitted to the hospital on 1/15 complaining of abdominal pain. The attending physician requested an upper GI series and laboratory evaluation of CBC and UA. The x-ray revealed possible cholelithiasis, and the UA showed an increased white blood cell count. The patient was taken to surgery for an exploratory laparoscopy, and a ruptured appendix was discovered. The chief complaint was:

    a. Ruptured appendix

    b. Exploratory laparoscopy

    c. Abdominal pain

    d. Cholelithiasis

62. All documentation entered in the medical record relating to the patient's diagnosis and treatment is considered as this type of data:

    a. Clinical

    b. Identification

    c. Secondary

    d. Financial

63. What type of data is exemplified by the insured party's member identification number?

    a. Demographic data

    b. Clinical data

    c. Certification data

    d. Financial data

64. Which part of the problem-oriented medical record is used by many facilities that have not adopted the whole problem-oriented format?

    a. Problem list as an index

    b. Initial plan

    c. SOAP form of progress notes

    d. Database

65. Whereas the focus of inpatient data collection is on the principal diagnosis, the focus of outpatient data collection is on:

    a. Reason for admission

    b. Reason for encounter

    c. Discharge diagnosis

    d. Activities of daily living

66. Mildred Smith was admitted from an acute-care hospital to a nursing facility with the following information: "Patient is being admitted for organic brain syndrome." Underneath the diagnosis, her medical information along with her rehabilitation potential were also listed. On which form is this information documented?

    a. Transfer or referral

    b. Release of information

    c. Patient rights acknowledgement

    d. Admitting physical evaluation

67. According to the Joint Commission Accreditation Standards, which document must be placed in the patient's record before a surgical procedure may be performed?

    a. Admission record

    b. Physician's order

    c. Report of history and physical examination

    d. Discharge summary

68. Bob Smith was admitted to Mercy Hospital on June 21. The physical examination was completed on June 23. According to Joint Commission standards, which statement applies to this situation?

    a. The record is not in compliance because the physical examination must be completed within 24 hours of admission.

    b. The record is not in compliance because the physical examination must be completed within 48 hours of admission.

    c. The record is in compliance because the physical examination must be completed within 48 hours of admission.

    d. The record is in compliance because the physical examination was completed within 72 hours of admission.

69. A health record with deficiencies that is not complete within the timeframe specified in the medical staff rules and regulations is called a(n):

    a. Suspended record

    b. Delinquent record

    c. Pending record

    d. Illegal record

70. The _____ may contain information about diseases among relatives in which heredity may play a role.

    a. Physical examination

    b. History

    c. Laboratory report

    d. Administrative data

Domain IV *Compliance*

71. To comply with Joint Commission standards, the HIM director wants to ensure that history and physical examinations are documented in the patient's health record no later than 24 hours after admission. Which of the following would be the *best* way to ensure the completeness of health records?

    a. Retrospectively review each patient's medical record to make sure history and physicals are present.

    b. Review each patient's medical record concurrently to make sure history and physicals are present and meet the accreditation standards.

    c. Establish a process to review medical records immediately on discharge.

    d. Do a review of records for all patients discharged in the previous 60 days.

72. Medical record completion compliance is a problem at Community Hospital. The number of incomplete charts often exceeds the standard set by the Joint Commission, risking a type I violation. Previous HIM committee chairpersons tried multiple methods to improve compliance, including suspension of privileges and deactivating the parking garage keycard of any physician in poor standing. To improve compliance, which of the following would be the next step to overcome noncompliance?

    a. Discuss the problem with the hospital CEO.

    b. Call the Joint Commission.

    c. Contact other hospitals to see what methods they use to ensure compliance.

    d. Drop the issue because noncompliance is always a problem.

73. How do accreditation organizations such as the Joint Commission use the health record?

    a. To serve as a source for case study information

    b. To determine whether the documentation supports the provider's claim for reimbursement

    c. To provide healthcare services

    d. To determine whether standards of care are being met

74. Valley High, a skilled nursing facility, wants to become certified to take part in federal government reimbursement programs such as Medicare. What standards must the facility meet in order to become certified for these programs?

    a. Joint Commission Accreditation Standards

    b. Accreditation Association for Ambulatory Healthcare Standards

    c. Conditions of Participation

    d. Outcomes and Assessment Information Set

75. What is the *best* source of documentation to determine the size of a removed malignant lesion?

    a. Pathology report

    b. Post–acute care unit record

    c. Operative report

    d. Physical examination

76. This document includes a microscopic description of tissue excised during surgery:

    a. Recovery room record

    b. Pathology report

    c. Operative report

    d. Discharge summary

77. When the physician does not specify the method used to remove a lesion during an endoscopy, what is the appropriate procedure?

    a. Assign the removal by snare technique code.

    b. Assign the removal by hot biopsy forceps code.

    c. Assign the ablation code.

    d. Query the physician as to the method used.

78. The Medicare Modernization Act of 2003 (MMA) launched a Medicare payment and recovery demonstration project that would later develop into recovery audit contractors (RACs) serving as a means to ensure correct payments under Medicare. During the demonstration program, the contractors were able to identify _____ of dollars in improper payments.

    a. Hundreds

    b. Thousands

    c. Millions

    d. Billions

79. Corporate compliance programs were released by the OIG for hospitals to develop and implement their own compliance programs. All of the following *except* _____ are basic elements of a corporate compliance program.

    a. Designation of a Chief Compliance Officer

    b. Implementation of regular and effective education and training programs for all employees

    c. Medical staff appointee for documentation compliance

    d. The use of audits or other evaluation techniques to monitor compliance

80. Which of the following programs has been in place in hospitals for years and has been required by the Medicare and Medicaid programs and accreditation standards?

    a. Internal DRG audits

    b. Peer review

    c. Managed care

    d. Quality improvement

81. Each year the OIG develops a work plan that details areas of compliance it will be investigating for that year. What is the expectation of the hospital in relation to the OIG work plan?

    a. Hospitals are required to follow the same work plan and deploy audits based on that work plan.

    b. Hospitals should plan their compliance and auditing projects around the OIG work plan to ensure they are in compliance with the target areas in the plan.

    c. Hospitals must not develop their audits based on the OIG work plan; rather, they must develop their own and look for high-risk areas that need improvement.

    d. Hospitals must use the plan developed by their state hospital association that is specific to state laws and compliance activities.

82. HIM coding professionals and the organizations that employ them have the responsibility to not tolerate behavior that adversely affects data quality. Which of the following is an example of behavior that should *not* be tolerated?

    a. Assign codes to an incomplete record with organizational policies in place to ensure codes are reviewed after the records are complete.

    b. Follow-up on and monitor identified problems.

    c. Evaluate and trend diagnoses and procedure code selections.

    d. Report data quality review results to organizational leadership, compliance staff, and the medical staff.

83. As recommended by AHIMA, HIM compliance policies and procedures should ensure all of the following *except:*

    a. Compensation for coders and consultants does not provide any financial incentive to code claims improperly

    b. The proper selection and sequencing of diagnoses codes

    c. Proper and timely documentation obtained before and after billing

    d The correct application of official coding rules and guidelines

84. An individual stole and used another person's insurance information to obtain medical care. This action would be considered:

    a. Violation of bioethics

    b. Fraud and abuse

    c. Medical identity theft

    d. Abuse

Domain V Information Technologies

85. A hospital HIM department wants to purchase an electronic system that records the location of health records removed from the filing system and documents the date of their return to the HIM department. Which of the following electronic systems would fulfill this purpose?

    a. Chart deficiency system

    b. Chart tracking system

    c. Chart abstracting system

    d. Chart encoder

86. What does an audit trail check for?

    a. Unauthorized access to a system

    b. Loss of data

    c. Presence of a virus

    d. Successful completion of a backup

87. An individual designated as an inpatient coder may have access to an electronic medical record to code the record. Under what access security mechanism is the coder allowed access to the system?

    a. Role-based

    b. User-based

    c. Context-based

    d. Situation-based

88. What software will prompt the user through a variety of questions and choices based on the clinical terminology entered to assist the coder in selecting the most appropriate code?

    a. Logic-based encoder

    b. Automated code book

    c. Speech recognition

    d. Natural-language processing

89. The technology commonly used for automated claims processing (sending bills directly to third-party payers) is:

    a. Optical character recognition

    b. Bar coding

    c. Neural networks

    d. Electronic data interchange

90. A software interface is a:

    a. Device to enter data

    b. Protocol for describing data

    c. Program to exchange data

    d. Standard vocabulary

91. A system that provides alerts and reminders to clinicians is a(n):

    a. Clinical decision support system

    b. Electronic data interchange

    c. Point of care charting system

    d. Knowledge database

92. A coder needs to locate electronic health records of a patient across a health information exchange (HIE). What tool(s) should the coder use?

    a. Certification

    b. Identity-matching algorithm and record locator service

    c. Interoperability and certification

    d. Meaningful use

Domain VI *Confidentiality and Privacy*

93. A hospital receives a valid request from a patient for copies of his or her medical records. The HIM clerk who is preparing the records removes copies of the patient's records from another hospital where the patient was previously treated. According to HIPAA regulations, was this action correct?

    a. Yes; HIPAA only requires that current records be produced for the patient.

    b. Yes; this is hospital policy over which HIPAA has no control.

    c. No; the records from the previous hospital are considered part of the designated record set and should be given to the patient.

    d. No; the records from the previous hospital are not included in the designated record set but should be released anyway.

94. A patient requests copies of her personal health information on CD. When the patient goes home, she finds that she cannot read the CD on her computer. The patient then requests the hospital to provide the medical records in paper format. How should the hospital respond?

    a. Provide the medical records in paper format

    b. Burn another CD because this is hospital policy

    c. Provide the patient with both paper and CD copies of the medical record

    d. Review the CD copies with the patient on a hospital computer

95. Which of the following definitions *best* describes the concept of confidentiality?

    a. The right of individuals to control access to their personal health information

    b. The protection of healthcare information from damage, loss, and unauthorized alteration

    c. The expectation that personal information shared by an individual with a healthcare provider during the course of care will be used only for its intended purpose

    d. The expectation that only individuals with the appropriate authority will be allowed to access healthcare information

96. The release of information function requires the HIM professional to have knowledge of:

    a. Clinical coding principles

    b. Database development

    c. Federal and state confidentiality laws

    d. Human resource management

97. The Medical Record Committee is reviewing the privacy policies for a large outpatient clinic. One of the members of the committee remarks that he feels the clinic's practice of calling out a patient's full name in the waiting room is not in compliance with HIPAA regulations and that only the patient's first name should be used. Other committee members disagree with this assessment. What should the HIM director advise the committee?

    a. HIPAA does not allow a patient's name to be announced in a waiting room.

    b. There is no HIPAA violation for announcing a patient's name, but the committee may want to consider implementing practices that might reduce this practice.

    c. HIPAA allows only the use of the patient's first name.

    d. HIPAA requires that patients be given numbers and only the number be announced.

98. The right of an individual to keep information about himself or herself from being disclosed to anyone is a definition of:

    a. Confidentiality

    b. Privacy

    c. Integrity

    d. Security

99. The HIM manager is concerned about whether the data transmitted across the hospital network is altered during the transmission. The concept that concerns the HIM manager is:

    a. Admissibility

    b. Disclosures

    c. Availability

    d. Data integrity

100. The CIA of security includes confidentiality, data integrity, and data _____.

    a. Accessibility

    b. Authentication

    c. Accuracy

    d. Availability

EXAM 2

Domain I *Clinical Classification Systems*

1. Identify the correct sequence and ICD-9-CM diagnosis code(s) for a patient with a scar on the right hand secondary to a laceration sustained two years ago.

   a. 709.2

   b. 906.1

   c. 709.2, 906.1

   d. 906.1, 709.2

2. Identify the correct sequence and ICD-9-CM diagnosis code(s) for a patient with dysphasia secondary to old cerebrovascular accident sustained one year ago.

   a. 787.20, 438.12

   b. 784.59, 438.12

   c. 438.12

   d. 787.20, 438.89

3. Identify the correct ICD-9-CM diagnosis code(s) for a patient with nausea, vomiting, and gastroenteritis.

   a. 558.9

   b. 787.01, 558.9

   c. 787.02, 787.03, 558.9

   d. 787.01, 558.41

4. Identify the correct ICD-9-CM diagnosis code for a patient with an elevated prostate-specific antigen (PSA) test result.

   a. 796.4

   b. 790.6

   c. 792.9

   d. 790.93

5. Identify the correct ICD-9-CM diagnosis code(s) for a patient with near-syncope event and nausea.

   a. 780.2

   b. 780.2, 787.02

   c. 780.2, 787.01

   d. 780.4, 787.02

6. Identify the correct ICD-9-CM diagnosis code(s) for a patient with an abnormal glucose tolerance test.

   a. 790.29

   b. 790.21

   c. 790.21, 790.29

   d. 790.22

7. Identify the correct ICD-9-CM diagnosis code(s) for a patient with pneumonia and persistent cough.

   a. 786.2, 490

   b. 486, 786.2

   c. 486

   d. 481

8. Identify the correct ICD-9-CM diagnosis code(s) for a patient with seizures; epilepsy ruled out.

   a. 780.39

   b. 345.9

   c. 780.39, 345.9

   d. 345.90

9. Identify the correct ICD-9-CM diagnosis code for a male patient with stress urinary incontinence.

   a. 625.6

   b. 788.30

   c. 788.32

   d. 788.39

10. Identify the correct ICD-9-CM diagnosis code(s) for a patient with right lower quadrant abdominal pain with nausea, vomiting, and diarrhea.

    a. 789.03

    b. 789.03, 787.02, 787.03, 787.91

    c. 789.03, 787.91

    d. 789.03, 787.01, 787.91

11. Identify the punctuation mark that is used to supplement words or explanatory information that may or may not be present in the statement of a diagnosis or procedure in ICD-9-CM coding. The punctuation does not affect the code number assigned to the case. The punctuation is considered a nonessential modifier, and all three volumes of ICD-9-CM use them.

    a. Parentheses ( )

    b. Square brackets [ ]

    c. Slanted brackets *[ ]*

    d. Braces { }

12. Identify the correct ICD-9-CM diagnosis code for a patient with anterolateral wall myocardial infarction, initial episode.

    a. 410.11

    b. 410.01

    c. 410.02

    d. 410.12

13. Identify the correct ICD-9-CM diagnosis code(s) and sequence for a patient with disseminated candidiasis secondary to AIDS-like syndrome.

    a. 042, 112.5, V01.79

    b. 112.5, 042

    c. 042, 112.5, V08

    d. 042, 112.5

14. Identify the correct ICD-9-CM diagnosis code(s) and proper sequencing for urinary tract infection due to *E. coli.*

    a. 599.0

    b. 599.0, 041.49

    c. 041.49

    d. 041.49, 599.0

15. Identify the correct ICD-9-CM diagnosis codes and sequence for a patient who was admitted to the outpatient chemotherapy floor for acute lymphocytic leukemia. During the procedure, the patient developed severe nausea with vomiting and was treated with medications.

    a. 204.00, 787.01, V58.11

    b. V58.11, 204.00, 787.01

    c. V58.11, 204.00

    d. 204.22, 787.01

16. Identify the correct ICD-9-CM diagnosis codes for metastatic carcinoma of the colon to the lung.

    a. 153.9, 162.9

    b. 197.0, 153.9

    c. 153.9, 197.0

    d. 153.9, 239.1

17. Identify the correct ICD-9-CM diagnosis code(s) for a patient with sepsis due to *Staphylococcus aureus* septicemia.

    a. 038.11, 995.91

    b. 995.91, 038.11

    c. 038.11

    d. 038.11, 995.92

18. Identify the ICD-9-CM diagnosis code(s) for uncontrolled Type II diabetes mellitus; mild malnutrition.

    a. 250.02

    b. 250.01, 263.1

    c. 250.02, 263.1

    d. 250.01, 263.0

19. Identify the ICD-9-CM diagnosis code(s) for neutropenic fever.

    a. 288.00

    b. 288.00, 780.60

    c. 288.01

    d. 288.00, 780.61

20. Mr. Smith is seen in his primary care physician's office for his annual physical examination. He has a digital rectal examination and is given three small cards to take home and return with fecal samples to screen for colorectal cancer. Assign the appropriate CPT code to report this occult blood sampling.

    a. 82270

    b. 82271

    c. 82272

    d. 82274

21. Category II codes cover all but one of the following topics. Which is *not* addressed by Category II codes?

    a. Patient management

    b. New technology

    c. Therapeutic, preventative, or other interventions

    d. Patient safety

22. Per CPT guidelines, a separate procedure is:

    a. Coded when it is performed as part of another, larger procedure

    b. Considered to be an integral part of another, larger service

    c. Never coded under any circumstance

    d. Both a and b

23. CPT was developed and is maintained by:

    a. CMS

    b. AMA

    c. Cooperating parties

    d. WHO

24. The codes in the musculoskeletal section of CPT may be used by:

    a. Orthopedic surgeons only

    b. Orthopedic surgeons and emergency department physicians

    c. Any physician

    d. Orthopedic surgeons and neurosurgeons

25. Observation E/M codes (99218–99220) are used in physician billing when:

    a. A patient is admitted and discharged on the same date.

    b. A patient is admitted for routine nursing care following surgery.

    c. A patient does not meet admission criteria.

    d. A patient is referred to a designated observation status.

26. Documentation in the history of use of drugs, alcohol, and tobacco is considered as part of the:

    a. Past medical history

    b. Social history

    c. Systems review

    d. History of present illness

27. Tissue transplanted from one individual to another of the same species, but different genotype is called a(n):

    a. Autograft

    b. Xenograft

    c. Allograft or allogeneic graft

    d. Heterograft

28. Mohs micrographic surgery involves the surgeon acting as:

    a. Both plastic surgeon and general surgeon

    b. Both surgeon and pathologist

    c. Both plastic surgeon and dermatologist

    d. Both dermatologist and pathologist

29. If an orthopedic surgeon attempted to reduce a fracture but was unsuccessful in obtaining acceptable alignment, what type of code should be assigned for the procedure?

    a. A "with manipulation" code

    b. A "without manipulation" code

    c. An unlisted procedure code

    d. An E/M code only

30. Identify the correct CPT procedure code for incision and drainage of infected shoulder bursa.

    a. 10060

    b. 10140

    c. 23030

    d. 23031

31. In coding arterial catheterizations, when the tip of the catheter is manipulated from the insertion into the aorta and then out into another artery, this is called:

    a. Selective catheterization

    b. Nonselective catheterization

    c. Manipulative catheterization

    d. Radical catheterization

32. When coding a selective catheterization in CPT, how are codes assigned?

    a. One code for each vessel entered

    b. One code for the point of entry vessel

    c. One code for the final vessel entered

    d. One code for the vessel of entry and one for the final vessel, with intervening vessels not coded

Domain II *Reimbursement Methodologies*

33. How does Medicare or other third-party payers determine whether the patient has medical necessity for the tests, procedures, or treatment billed on a claim form?

    a. By requesting the medical record for each service provided

    b. By reviewing all the diagnosis codes assigned to explain the reasons the services were provided

    c. By reviewing all physician orders

    d. By reviewing the discharge summary and history and physical report of the patient over the last year

34. What is the name of the organization that develops the billing form that hospitals are required to use?

    a. American Academy of Billing Forms (AABF)

    b. National Uniform Billing Committee (NUBC)

    c. National Uniform Claims Committee (NUCC)

    d. American Billing and Claims Academy (ABCA)

35. What healthcare organizations collect UHDDS data?

    a. All outpatient settings including physician clinics and ambulatory surgical centers

    b. All outpatient settings including cancer centers, independent testing facilities, and nursing homes

    c. All non outpatient settings including acute care, short-term care, long-term care, and psychiatric hospitals; home health agencies; rehabilitation facilities; and nursing homes

    d. All inpatient settings and outpatient settings with a focus on ambulatory surgical centers

36. What was the goal of the MS-DRG system?

    a. To improve Medicare's capability to recognize severity of illness in its inpatient hospital payments. The new system is projected to increase payments to hospitals for services provided to sicker patients and decrease payments for treating less severely ill patients.

    b. To improve Medicare's capability to recognize poor quality of care and pay hospitals on an incentive grid that allows hospitals to be paid by performance.

    c. To improve Medicare's capability to recognize groups of data by patient populations, which will further allow Medicare to adjust the hospitals wage indexes based on the data. This adjustment will be a system to pay hospitals fairly across all geographic locations.

    d. To improve Medicare's capability to recognize practice patterns among hospitals that are inappropriately optimizing payments by keeping patients in the hospital longer than the median length of stay.

37. What is the basic formula for calculating each MS-DRG hospital payment?

    a. Hospital payment = DRG relative weight $\times$ hospital base rate

    b. Hospital payment = DRG relative weight $\times$ hospital base rate $-$ 1

    c. Hospital payment = DRG relative weight / hospital base rate $+$ 1

    d. Hospital payment = DRG relative weight / hospital base rate

38. What are the possible "add-on" payments that a hospital could receive in addition to the basic Medicare DRG payment?

    a. Additional payments may be made for locum tenens, increased emergency room services, stays over the average length of stay, and cost outlier cases.

    b. Additional payments may be made to critical access hospitals, for higher-than-normal volumes, unexpected hospital emergencies, and cost outlier cases.

    c. Additional payments may be made for increased emergency room services, critical access hospitals, increased labor costs, and cost outlier cases.

    d. Additional payments may be made to disproportionate share hospitals for indirect medical education, new technologies, and cost outlier cases.

39. What is the name of the national program to detect and correct improper payments in the Medicare Fee-for-Service (FFS) program?

    a. Medicare administrative contractors (MACs)

    b. Recovery audit contractors (RACs)

    c. Comprehensive error rate testing (CERT)

    d. Fiscal intermediaries (FIs)

40. What is the maximum number of procedure codes that can appear on a UB-04 institutional claim form via electronic transmission?

    a. 6

    b. 9

    c. 15

    d. 25

41. Which answer *fails* to provide a requirement for assignment of the MS-DRG?

    a. Diagnoses and procedures (principal and secondary)

    b. Attending and consulting physicians

    c. Presence of major or other complications and comorbidities (MCC or CC)

    d. Discharge disposition or status

42. What is the maximum number of diagnosis codes that can appear on the UB-04 paper claim form locator 67 for a hospital inpatient principal and secondary diagnoses?

    a. 35

    b. 25

    c. 18

    d. 9

43. Which of the following situations would be identified by the NCCI edits?

    a. Determining the MS-DRG

    b. Billing for two services that are prohibited from being billed on the same day

    c. Whether data submitted electronically were successfully submitted

    d. Receiving the remittance advice

44. A hospital needs to know how much Medicare paid on a claim so they can bill the secondary insurance. What should the hospital refer to?

    a. Explanation of benefits

    b. Medicare Summary Notice

    c. Remittance advice

    d. Coordination of benefits

45. A patient has two health insurance policies: Medicare and a Medicare supplement. Which of the following statements is true?

    a. The patient receives any monies paid by the insurance companies over and above the charges.

    b. Monies paid to the healthcare provider cannot exceed charges.

    c. The decision on which company is primary is based on remittance advice.

    d. The patient should not have a Medicare supplement.

46. The purpose of a physician query is to:

    a. Identify the MS-DRG

    b. Identify the principal diagnosis

    c. Improve documentation for patient care and proper reimbursement

    d. Increase reimbursement as form of optimization

47. What is it called when a Medicare hospital inpatient admission results in exceptionally high costs when compared to other cases in the same DRG?

    a. Rate increase

    b. Charge outlier

    c. Cost outlier

    d. Day outlier

48. What is a chargemaster?

    a. Cost-sharing in which the policy or certificate holder pays a preestablished percentage of eligible expenses after the deductible has been met

    b. A plan that converts the organization's goals and objectives into targets for revenue and spending

    c. A financial management form that contains information about the organization's charges for the healthcare services it provides to patients

    d. Charged amounts that are billed as costs by an organization to the current year's activities of operation

49. A fee schedule is:

    a. Developed by third-party payers and includes a list of healthcare services, procedures, and charges associated with each

    b. Developed by providers and includes a list of healthcare services provided to a patient

    c. Developed by third-party payers and includes a list of healthcare services provided to a patient

    d. Developed by providers and lists charge codes

50. The provider or supplier is prohibited from holding the patient responsible for charges in excess of the Medicare fee schedule. This is called:

   a. Accept assignment

   b. Balance billing

   c. Charge capture

   d. Inducement

51. If a provider believes a service may be denied by Medicare because it could be considered unnecessary, the provider must notify the patient before the treatment begins by using a(n):

   a. Advance beneficiary notice (ABN)

   b. Advance notice of coverage (ANC)

   c. Notice of payment (NOP)

   d. Consent for payment (CFP)

52. Assignment of benefits is a contract between a physician and Medicare in which the physician agrees to bill Medicare directly for covered services and the beneficiary only for _____ and to accept the Medicare payment as payment in full.

   a. Coinsurance or deductible

   b. Deductible only

   c. Coinsurance only

   d. Balance of charges

53. A provision of the law that established the resource-based relative value scale (RBRVS) stipulates that refinements to relative value units (RVUs) must maintain:

   a. Moderate rate increases

   b. Market basket increases

   c. Budget neutrality

   d. Sustainable growth rate

54. Reimbursement for healthcare services is dependent on patients having a(n):

   a. Attending physician

   b. Insurance benefit

   c. Explanation of benefits

   d. Qualified provider

55. Health insurance for spouses, children, or both is known as:

   a. Dependent (family) coverage

   b. Individual (single) coverage

   c. Group coverage

   d. Inclusive coverage

Domain III *Health Records and Data Content*

56. Documentation regarding a patient's marital status; dietary, sleep, and exercise patterns; and use of coffee, tobacco, alcohol, and other drugs may be found in the:

    a. Physical examination record

    b. History record

    c. Operative report

    d. Radiological report

57. A patient with known COPD and hypertension under treatment was admitted to the hospital with symptoms of a lower abdominal pain. He undergoes a laparoscopic appendectomy and develops a fever. The patient was subsequently discharged from the hospital with a principal diagnosis of acute appendicitis and secondary diagnoses of postoperative infection, COPD, and hypertension. Which of the following diagnoses should *not* be tagged as POA?

    a. Postoperative infection

    b. Appendicitis

    c. COPD

    d. Hypertension

58. Which of the following would *not* be found in a medical history?

    a. Chief complaint

    b. Vital signs

    c. Present illness

    d. Review of systems

59. Which of the following reports includes names of the surgeon and assistants, date, duration and description of the procedure, and any specimens removed?

    a. Operative report

    b. Anesthesia report

    c. Pathology report

    d. Laboratory report

60. Identify the acute-care record report where the following information would be found: The patient is a well-developed, obese male who does not appear to be in any distress but has considerable problem with mobility. He has difficulty rising up from a chair, and he uses a cane to ambulate. VITAL SIGNS: His blood pressure today is 158/86, pulse is 80 per minute, weight is 204 pounds (which is 13 pounds below what he weighed in the previous month). He has no pallor. He has rather pronounced shaking of his arms, which he claims is not new. NECK: Showed no jugular venous distension. HEART: Very irregular. LUNGS: Clear. EXTREMITIES: Edema of both legs.

    a. Discharge summary

    b. Medical history

    c. Medical laboratory report

    d. Physical examination

61. Identify the acute-care record report where the following information would be found: Gross Description: Received fresh designated left lacrimal gland is a single, unoriented, irregular, tan-pink portion of soft tissue measuring $0.8 \times 0.6 \times 0.1$ cm, which is submitted entirely intact in one cassette.

    a. Medical history

    b. Medical laboratory report

    c. Pathology report

    d. Physical examination

62. Which organization developed the first hospital standardization program?

    a. Joint Commission

    b. American Osteopathic Association

    c. American College of Surgeons

    d. American Association of Medical Colleges

63. The hospital is revising its policy on medical record documentation. Currently, all entries in the medical record must be legible, complete, dated, and signed. The committee chairperson wants to add that, in addition, all entries must have the time noted. However, another clinician suggests that adding the time of notation is difficult and rarely may be correct since personal watches and hospital clocks may not be coordinated. Another committee member agrees and says only electronic documentation needs a time stamp. Given this discussion, which of the following might the HIM director suggest?

    a. Suggest that only hospital clock time be noted in clinical documentation

    b. Suggest that only electronic documentation have time noted

    c. Inform the committee that according to the Medicare Conditions of Participation, all documentation must be authenticated and dated

    d. Inform the committee that according to the Medicare Conditions of Participation, only medication orders must include date and time

64. When correcting erroneous information in a health record, which of the following is *not* appropriate?

    a. Print "error" above the entry

    b. Enter the correction in chronological sequence

    c. Add the reason for the change

    d. Use black pen to obliterate the entry

65. Community Hospital implemented a clinical document improvement (CDI) program six months ago. The goal of the program was to improve clinical documentation to support quality of care, data quality, and HIM coding accuracy. Which of the following would be the *best* to ensure that everyone understands the importance of this program?

    a. Request that the CEO write a memorandum to all hospital staff.

    b. Give the chairperson of the CDI committee authority to fire employees who do not improve their clinical documentation.

    c. Include ancillary clinical and medical staff in the process.

    d. Request a letter from the Joint Commission.

66. In a routine health record quantitative analysis review, it was found that a physician dictated a discharge summary on 1/26/20XX. The patient, however, was discharged two days later. In this case, what would be the best course of action?

    a. Request that the physician dictate another discharge summary.

    b. Have the record analyst note the date discrepancy.

    c. Request the physician dictate an addendum to the discharge summary.

    d. File the record as complete because the discharge summary includes all of the pertinent patient information.

67. During an audit of health records, the HIM director finds that transcribed reports are being changed by the author up to a week after initial transcription. The director is concerned that changes occurring this long after transcription jeopardize the legal principle that documentation must occur near the time of the event. To remedy this situation, the HIM director should recommend which of the following?

    a. Immediately stop the practice of changing transcribed reports.

    b. Develop a facility policy that defines the acceptable period of time allowed for a transcribed document to remain in draft form.

    c. Conduct a verification audit.

    d. Alert hospital legal counsel of the practice.

68. During a review of documentation practices, the HIM director finds that nurses are routinely using the copy-and-paste function of the hospital's new EHR system for documenting nursing notes. In some cases, nurses are copying and pasting the objective data from the lab system and intake–output records as well as the patient's subjective complaints and symptoms originally documented by another practitioner. Which of the following should the HIM director do to ensure the nurses are following acceptable documentation practices?

    a. Inform the nurses that "copy and paste" is not acceptable and to stop this practice immediately.

    b. Determine how many nurses are involved in this practice.

    c. Institute an in-service training session on documentation practices.

    d. Develop policies and procedures related to cutting, copying, and pasting documentation in the EHR system.

69. Who is responsible for writing and signing discharge summaries and discharge instructions?

    a. Attending physician

    b. Head nurse

    c. Primary physician

    d. Admitting nurse

70. Where would a coder who needed to locate the histology of a tissue sample most likely find this information?

    a. Pathology report

    b. Progress notes

    c. Nurse's notes

    d. Operative report

Domain IV *Compliance*

71. An HIM professional's ethical obligations:

    a. Apply regardless of employment site

    b. Are limited to the employer

    c. Apply to only the patient

    d. Are limited to the employer and patient

72. Which of the following is the concept of the right of an individual to be left alone?

    a. Privacy

    b. Bioethics

    c. Security

    d. Confidentiality

73 What should be done when the HIM department's error or accuracy rate is deemed unacceptable?

    a. A corrective action should be taken.

    b. The problem should be treated as an isolated incident.

    c. The formula for determining the rate may need to be adjusted.

    d. Re-audit the problem area.

74 Statements that define the performance expectations and structures or processes that must be in place are:

    a. Rules

    b. Policies

    c. Guidelines

    d. Standards

75 In an EHR, what is the risk of copying and pasting?

    a. Reduction in the time required to document

    b. The system not recording who entered the data

    c. Quicker overall system response time

    d. System thinking that the original documenter recorded the note

76 How are amendments handled in an EHR?

    a. Automatically appended to the original note; no additional signature is required.

    b. Amendments must be entered by the same person as the original note.

    c. Amendments cannot be entered after 24 hours of the event's occurrence.

    d. The amendment must have a separate signature, date, and time.

77. The Privacy Rule establishes that a patient has the right of access to inspect and obtain a copy of his or her PHI:

    a. For as long as it is maintained

    b. For six years

    c. Forever

    d. For 12 months

78. HIPAA regulations:

    a. Never preempt state statutes

    b. Always preempt state statutes

    c. Preempt less-strict state statutes where they exist

    d. Preempt stricter state statutes where they exist

79 The Privacy Rule applies to:

    a. All covered entities involved with transmitting or performing any electronic transactions specified in the act

    b. Healthcare providers only

    c. Only healthcare providers that receive Medicare reimbursement

    d. Only entities funded by the federal government

80. Which of the following is the concept responsible for limiting disclosure of private matters including the responsibility to use, disclose, or release such information only with the knowledge and consent of the individual?

    a. Privacy

    b. Bioethics

    c. Security

    d. Confidentiality

81. Which of the following is *not* an accepted accrediting body for behavioral healthcare organizations?

    a. American Psychological Association

    b. Joint Commission

    c. Commission on Accreditation of Rehabilitation Facilities

    d. National Committee for Quality Assurance

82. What type of standard establishes methods for creating unique designations for individual patients, healthcare professionals, healthcare provider organizations, and healthcare vendors and suppliers?

    a. Vocabulary standard

    b. Identifier standard

    c. Structure and content standard

    d. Security standard

83. What type of organization works under contract with the CMS to conduct Medicare and Medicaid certification surveys for hospitals?

    a. Accreditation organizations

    b. Certification organizations

    c. State licensure agencies

    d. Conditions of participation agencies

84. Which of the following threatens the "need-to-know" principle?

    a. Backdating progress notes

    b. Blanket authorization

    c. HIPAA regulations

    d. Surgical consent

Domain V *Information Technologies*

85. A hospital is planning on allowing coding professionals to work at home. The hospital is in the process of identifying strategies to minimize the security risks associated with this practice. Which of the following would be *best* to ensure that data breaches are minimized when the home computer is unattended?

    a. User name and password

    b. Automatic session terminations

    c. Cable locks

    d. Encryption

86. A coding analyst consistently enters the wrong code for patient gender in the electronic billing system. What security measures should be in place to minimize this security breach?

    a. Access controls

    b. Audit trail

    c. Edit checks

    d. Password controls

87. Which of the following would be the *best* technique to ensure that registration clerks consistently use the correct notation for assigning admission date in an electronic health record (EHR)?

    a. Make admission date a required field

    b. Provide an input mask for entering data in the field

    c. Make admission date a numeric field

    d. Provide sufficient space for input of data

88. In hospitals, automated systems for registering patients and tracking their encounters are commonly known as _____ systems.

   a. MIS

   b. CDS

   c. ADT

   d. ABC

89. Which of the following provides organizations with the ability to access data from multiple databases and to combine the results into a single questions-and-reporting interface?

   a. Client-server computer

   b. Data warehouse

   c. Local area network

   d. Internet

90. The _____ is a type of coding that is a natural outgrowth of the EHR.

   a. Automated codebook

   b. Computer-assisted coding

   c. Logic-based encoder

   d. Decision support database

91. A(n) _____ is a computer software that assists in determining coding accuracy and reliability.

   a. Encoder

   b. Interface

   c. Diagnosis-related group

   d. Record locator service

92 The _____ uses expert or artificial intelligence software to automatically assign code numbers.

   a. Functional EHR

   b. NHIN

   c. NLP encoding system

   d. Grouper

Domain VI *Confidentiality and Privacy*

93. Data security policies and procedures should be reviewed at least:

   a. Semi annually

   b. Annually

   c. Every two years

   d. Quarterly

94. Which of the following ethical principles is being followed when an HIT professional ensures that patient information is only released to those who have a legal right to access it?

    a. Autonomy

    b. Beneficence

    c. Justice

    d. Nonmaleficence

95. Which of the following is a threat to data security?

    a. Encryption

    b. People

    c. Red flags

    d. Access controls

96. Under the HIPAA privacy standard, which of the following types of protected health information (PHI) must be specifically identified in an authorization?

    a. History and physical reports

    b. Operative reports

    c. Consultation reports

    d. Psychotherapy notes

97. What penalties can be enforced against a person or entity that willfully and knowingly violates the HIPAA Privacy Rule with the intent to sell, transfer, or use PHI for commercial advantage, personal gain, or malicious harm?

    a. A fine of not more than $10,000 only

    b. A fine of not more than $10,000, not more than one year in jail, or both

    c. A fine of not more than $5,000 only

    d. A fine of not more than $250,000, not more than 10 years in jail, or both

98. An HIT using her password can access and change data in the hospital's master patient index. A billing clerk, using his password, cannot perform the same function. Limiting the class of information and functions that can be performed by these two employees is managed by:

    a. Network controls

    b. Audit trails

    c. Administrative controls

    d. Access controls

99. An employee in the physical therapy department arrives early every morning to snoop through the clinical information system for potential information about neighbors and friends. What security mechanisms should be implemented to prevent this security breach?

    a. Audit controls

    b. Information access controls

    c. Facility access controls

    d. Workstation security

100. What should a hospital do when a state law requires more stringent privacy protection than the federal HIPAA privacy standard?

a. Ignore the state law and follow the HIPAA standard

b. Follow the state law and ignore the HIPAA standard

c. Comply with both the state law and the HIPAA standard

d. Ignore both the state law and the HIPAA standard and follow relevant accreditation standards

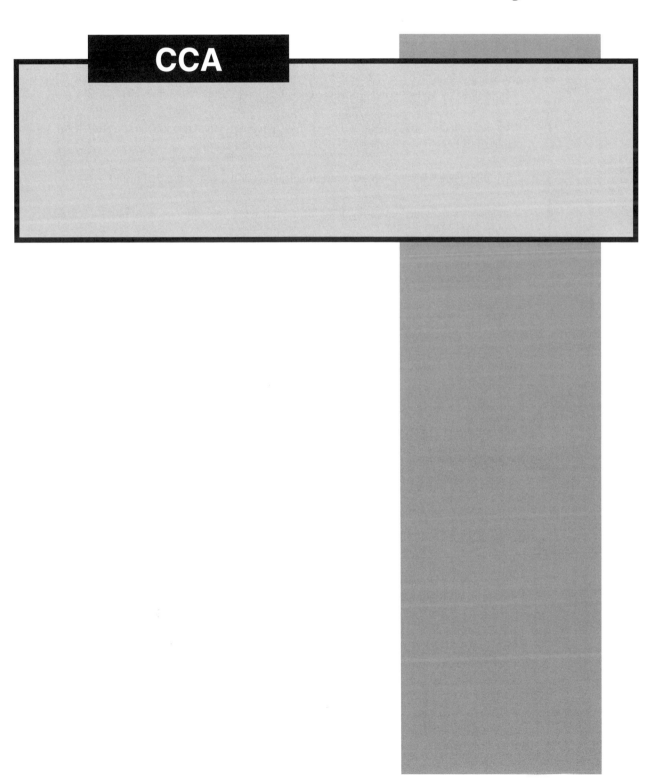

Answer Key

CCA

CCA Practice Questions

1. **a**   Index Carcinoma, in situ, see also Neoplasm, by site, in situ (Schraffenberger 2012, 94–95.)

2. **b**   Index Melanoma (malignant), shoulder. Melanoma is considered a malignant neoplasm and is referenced as such in the index of ICD-9-CM. The term "benign neoplasm" is considered a growth that does not invade adjacent structures or spread to distant sites but may displace or exert pressure on adjacent structures (Schraffenberger 2012, 94–95).

3. **b**   NCHS is responsible for updating the diagnosis classification (Volumes 1 and 2), and CMS is responsible for updating the procedure classification (Volume 3) (Johns 2011, 239).

4. **d**   The most specific codes in the ICD-9-CM system are found at the subclassification level (Johns 2011, 240).

5. **d**   Five-digit code numbers represent the subclassification level (Johns 2011, 240).

6. **c**   Categories are divided into subcategories. At this level, four-digit code numbers are used (Johns 2011, 240).

7. **d**   V codes are always alphanumeric codes. They are easy to identify because they begin with the alpha character V and follow with numeric digits (Johns 2011, 242).

8. **b**   E codes provide a means to describe environmental events, circumstances, and conditions as the cause of injury, poisoning, and other adverse effects (Johns 2011, 242).

9. **c**   ICD-9-CM Volume 3 contains the Tabular List and Alphabetic Index of procedures (Johns 2011, 243).

10. **c**   Index Lipoma, face. ICD-9-CM classifies neoplasms by system, organ, or site with the exception of neoplasms of the lymphatic and hematopoietic system, malignant melanomas of the skin, lipomas, common tumors of the bone, uterus, and ovary. Because of these exceptions, the Alphabetic Index must first be checked to determine whether a code has been assigned for that specific histology type (Schraffenberger 2012, 99–100).

11. **a**   Index Adenoma, adrenal (cortex). Index Syndrome, Conn. According to the Index in ICD-9-CM, except where otherwise indicated, the morphological varieties of adenoma should be coded by site as for "Neoplasm, benign" (Schraffenberger 2012, 100).

12. **a**   CPT is a comprehensive descriptive listing of terms and codes for reporting diagnostic and therapeutic procedures and medical services (Johns 2011, 255).

13. **c**   Index Contusion, cerebral—see Contusion, brain. Add a fifth digit of "2" for brief loss of consciousness. Cerebral contusions are often caused by a blow to the head. A cerebral contusion is a more severe injury involving a bruise of the brain with bleeding into the brain tissue, but without disruption of the brain's continuity. The loss of consciousness that occurs often lasts longer than that of a concussion. Codes for cerebral laceration and contusion range from 851.0 to 851.9, with fifth digits added to indicate whether a loss of consciousness or concussion occurred (Schraffenberger 2012, 359).

14. **d** The code selection is determined by measuring the greatest clinical diameter of the apparent lesion plus that margin required for complete excision (lesion diameter plus the most narrow margins required equals the excised diameter) (AMA 2012, 64).

15. **a** Complex closure includes the repair of wounds requiring more than layered closure, namely, scar revision, debridement, extensive undermining, stents, or retention sutures (AMA 2012c, 66).

16. **a** Subsequent admissions for retained products of conception following a spontaneous or legally induced abortion are assigned the appropriate code from category 634, spontaneous abortion, or 635, legally induced abortion, with a fifth digit of "1" (incomplete). This advice is appropriate even when the patient was discharged previously with a discharge diagnosis of complete abortion (Schraffenberger 2012, 264–266).

17. **c** The term "urosepsis" is a nonspecific term. If that is the only term documented, only code 599.0 should be assigned based on the default for the term in the ICD-9-CM index, in addition to the code for the causal organism, if known. Septicemia results from the entry of pathogens into the bloodstream. Symptoms include spiking fever, chills, and skin eruptions in the form of petechiae or purpura. Blood cultures are usually positive; however, a negative culture does not exclude the diagnosis of septicemia. Several other clinical indications and symptomology could indicate the diagnosis of septicemia. Only the physician can diagnose the condition based on clinical indications. Query the physician when the diagnosis is not clear to the coder (Schraffenberger 2012, 79–81, 251).

18. **c** If treatment is directed at the malignancy, designate the malignancy as the principal diagnosis. The only exception to this guideline is if a patient admission or encounter is solely for the administration of chemotherapy, immunotherapy, or radiation therapy, assign the appropriate V code as the first-listed or principal diagnosis and the diagnosis or problem for which the service is being performed as a secondary diagnosis (Schraffenberger 2012, 97–98).

19. **b** Gastroenteritis is characterized by diarrhea, nausea, and vomiting, and abdominal cramps. Codes for symptoms, signs, and ill-defined conditions from Chapter 16 of the CPT codebook are not to be used as the principal diagnosis when a related definitive diagnosis has been established. Patients can have several chronic conditions that coexist at the time of their hospital admission and qualify as additional diagnosis such as COPD and angina (Schraffenberger 2012, 66–68, 71–72, 236).

20. **c** When a primary malignancy has been previously excised or eradicated from its site and there is no further treatment directed to that site and there is no evidence of any existing primary malignancy, a code from category V10, personal history of malignant neoplasm, should be used to indicate the former site of the malignancy. Any mention of extension, invasion, or metastatic to another site is coded as a secondary malignant neoplasm to that site. The secondary site may be the principal, with the V10 code used as a secondary code (Schraffenberger 2012, 98).

21. **a** In the unusual instance when two or more diagnoses equally meet the criteria for principal diagnosis, as determined by the circumstances of admission, diagnostic workup, and the therapy provided, and the Alphabetic Index, Tabular List, or another coding guideline does not provide sequencing direction in such cases, any one of the diagnoses may be sequenced first (Schraffenberger 2012, 68–69).

22. **c** For reporting purposes the definition for "other diagnoses" is interpreted as additional conditions that affect patient care in terms of requiring: clinical evaluation, therapeutic treatment, diagnostic procedures, extended length of hospital stay, increased nursing care, and monitoring (Schraffenberger 2012, 71).

23. **c** A patient in status asthmaticus fails to respond to therapy administered during an asthmatic attack. This is a life-threatening condition that requires emergency care and likely hospitalization (Schraffenberger 2012, 222–223).

24. **d** Signs, symptoms, abnormal test results, or other reasons for the outpatient visit are used when a physician qualifies a diagnostic statement as "rule out" or other similar terms indicating uncertainty. In the outpatient setting the condition qualified in that statement should not be coded as if it existed. Rather, the condition should be coded to the highest degree of certainty, such as the sign or symptom the patient exhibits. In this case, assign the code 786.50, Chest pain NOS (Schraffenberger 2012, 339).

25. **c** For outpatient encounters for diagnostic tests that have been interpreted by a physician, and the final report is available at the time of coding, code any confirmed or definitive diagnosis(es) documented in the interpretation. Do not code related signs and symptoms as additional diagnosis. Note: This differs from the coding practice in the hospital inpatient setting regarding abnormal findings on test results (Schraffenberger 2012, 340–341).

26. **c** The disproportion was specified as cephalopelvic; thus the correct ICD-9-CM code is 653.41. Two codes are required for anesthesia: one for the planned vaginal delivery (01967) and an add-on code (01968) to describe anesthesia for cesarean delivery following planned vaginal delivery converted to cesarean. An instructional note guides the coder to use 01968 with 01967 (Schraffenberger 2012, 272–273; AMA 2012, 52).

27. **d** According to Central Office on ICD-9-CM, ICD-9-CM is not used to collect data about nursing care (Johns 2011, 239).

28. **d** According to Central Office on ICD-9-CM, ICD-9-CM is not used to identify supplies, products, and services used by patients (Johns 2011, 239).

29. **a** ICD-9-CM Volume 1 is known as the Tabular List and contains the numerical listing of codes that represent diseases and injuries (Johns 2011, 239).

30. **a** Follow instructions under the main term in the Alphabetic Index. Instructions in the index should be followed when determining which column to use in the neoplasm table. In this example, malignant is not a choice in the Alphabetic Index shown. Benign in category 216 indicates all of the diagnosis codes in this category are benign (Schraffenberger 2012, 95, 100).

31. **b** Code 434.91 is assigned when the diagnosis states stroke, cerebrovascular, or cerebrovascular accident (CVA) without further specification. The health record should be reviewed to make sure nothing more specific is available. Conditions resulting from an acute cerebrovascular disease, such as aphasia or hemiplegia, should be coded as well (Schraffenberger 2012, 198–199).

32. **a** Acute respiratory failure, code 518.81, may be assigned as a principal or secondary diagnosis depending on the circumstances of the inpatient admission. Chapter-specific coding guidelines (obstetrics, poisoning, HIV, newborn) provide specific sequencing direction. Respiratory failure may be listed as a secondary diagnosis. If respiratory failure occurs after admission, it may be listed as a secondary diagnosis (Schraffenberger 2012, 224–226).

33. **d**   Adverse effects can occur in situation in which medication is administered properly and prescribed correctly in both therapeutic and diagnostic procedures. An adverse effect can occur when everything is done correctly. The first-listed diagnosis is the manifestation or the nature of the adverse effect, such as the hematuria. Locate the drug in the Substance column of the Table of Drugs and Chemicals in the Alphabetic Index to Diseases. Select the E code for the drug from the Therapeutic Use column of the Table of Drugs and Chemicals. Use of the E code is mandatory when coding adverse effects (Schraffenberger 2012, 377–378).

34. **c**   Use a fifth digit of "1" to designate the first episode of care (regardless of facility site) for a newly diagnosed myocardial infarction. The fifth digit "1" is assigned regardless of the number of times a patient may be transferred during the initial episode of care (Schraffenberger 2012, 188).

35. **b**   The principal diagnosis determines the MDC assignment (Johns 2011, 322).

36. **a**   All claims involving inpatient admissions to general acute care hospitals or other facilities that are subject to law or regulation mandating collection of present on admission information. *Present on admission* (POA) is defined as present at the time the order for inpatient admission occurs. Conditions that develop during an outpatient encounter, including emergency department, observation, or outpatient surgery, are considered POA. Any condition that occurs after admission is not considered a POA condition (Schraffenberger 2012, 66).

37. **b**   A *complication* is a secondary condition that arises during hospitalization and is thought to increase the length of stay by at least one day for approximately 75% of the patients (Johns 2011, 322).

38. **b**   *Septicemia* generally refers to a systemic disease associated with the presence of pathological microorganisms or toxins in the blood, which can include bacteria, viruses, fungi, or other organisms. Code 038.11 is assigned for septicemia with *Staphylococcus aureus*. Because abdominal pain is a symptom of diverticulosis, only the diverticulitis of the colon (562.11) is coded (Schraffenberger 2012, 80).

39. **c**   When the primary malignant neoplasm previously removed by surgery or eradicated by radiotherapy or chemotherapy recurs, the primary malignant code for the site is assigned, unless the Alphabetic Index directs otherwise (Schraffenberger 2012, 106).

40. **a**   The ventral hernia is coded as the primary or first-listed diagnosis. The repair of the hernia is not coded because it was not performed; however, code 54.11 is assigned to describe the extent of the procedure, which is an exploratory laparotomy. The V64.3 is coded to indicate the cancelled procedure. Code 427.89 is also used to describe the bradycardia that the patient develops during the procedure (Schraffenberger 2012, 46–47).

41. **b**   *V codes* are diagnosis codes and indicate a reason for healthcare encounter (Schraffenberger 2012, 433).

42. **b**   The fracture is the principal diagnosis, with the contusions as a secondary diagnosis. The fracture is what required in the most treatment. Procedures for the reduction, debridement, and external fixation device would all need to be coded (Schraffenberger 2012, 354–355).

43. **d**   Begin with the main term Revision; pacemaker site; chest (Kuehn 2012, 27, 142).

44. **a**   Code 54401 is correct because the prosthesis is self-contained (Kuehn 2012, 27, 178).

45. **d** Modifier –24 is used for unrelated evaluation and management service by the same physician during a postoperative period (Kuehn 2012, 53).

46. **d** If the patient is admitted in withdrawal or if withdrawal develops after admission, the withdrawal code is designated as the principal diagnosis. The code for substance abuse or dependence is listed second (Schraffenberger 2012, 148).

47. **a** The anemia would be sequenced first based on principal diagnosis guidelines (Schraffenberger 2012, 64).

48. **d** The patient was admitted for the senile cataract and the procedures were completed for that condition. This follows the UHDDS guidelines for principle diagnosis selection. There is also no causal relationship given between the diabetes and the cataract, so 250.50 would be incorrect (Schraffenberger 2012, 122–123, 164).

49. **d** Patient was admitted for COPD, so this is listed as the principal diagnosis. Code 491.21 is used when the medical record includes documentation of COPD with acute exacerbation. ICD-9-CM presumes a cause-and-effect relationship and classifies chronic kidney disease with hypertension as hypertensive chronic kidney disease, code 403.91; however, the code also at category 403 directs the coder to also code the chronic renal failure 585.9 (Schraffenberger 2012, 182–184, 222–223).

50. **c** The closed reduction of the fracture is coded first, following principal procedure guidelines. The laceration repair is also coded. When more than one classification of wound repair is performed, all codes are reported, with the code for the most complicated procedure listed first (Kuehn 2012, 30–31, 111–112).

51. **c** A bronchoscopy with brushings and washings is considered a diagnostic bronchoscopy and not a biopsy. Code 31623 specifies brushings, and code 31622 is selected for washings (Kuehn 2012, 136–137).

52. **d** Modifiers are appended to the code to provide more information or to alert the payer that a payment change is required. Modifier –55 is used to identify the physician provided only postoperative care services for a particular procedure (Kuehn 2012, 292, 295).

53. **b** Index main term: Destruction, hemorrhoid, thermal. Thermal includes infrared coagulation (Kuehn 2012, 27, 163).

54. **c** A *logic-based encoder* prompts the user through a variety of questions and choices based on the clinical terminology entered. The coder selects the most accurate code for a service or condition (and any possible complications or comorbidities) (LaTour and Eichenwald Maki 2010, 400).

55. **a** Main term: Depression; subterm: recurrent with fifth digit of 3 for severe, without mention of psychotic behavior (Schraffenberger 2012, 143–145).

56. **c** Main term for procedure: Esophagoscopy; subterm: with closed biopsy (Schraffenberger 2012, 44–45).

57. **d** Codes for symptoms, signs, and ill-defined conditions are not to be used as the principal diagnosis when a related definitive diagnosis has been established. The flank pain would not be coded because it is a symptom of the calculus (Schraffenberger 2012, 67-68).

58. **c** Main term for diagnosis: Incontinence; subterm: stress. Main term for procedure: Suspension; subterm: urethra (Schraffenberger 2012, 10).

59. **c** Index the main term of Hernia repair; inguinal; incarcerated. The age of the patient and the fact that the hernia is not recurrent make the choice 49507. Providing information regarding insurance coverage is not a function of the discharge summary (Kuehn 2012, 27, 164–166).

60. **c** Begin with the main term of Hernia repair; incisional. The fact that the hernia is recurrent, done via a laparoscope, and is reducible makes the choice 49656. Notice that the use of mesh is included in the code (Kuehn 2012, 27, 164–166).

61. **b** Main term of Hysteroscopy; lysis; adhesions (Kuehn 2012, 27, 182–184).

62. **d** In the abdomen, peritoneum, and omentum subsection, the exploratory laparotomy is a separate procedure and should not be reported when it is part of a larger procedure. The code of 49000 is not reported because laparotomy is the approach to the surgery. The code 58720 includes bilateral so the modifier –50 is not necessary to report (Kuehn 2012, 163–164, 184).

63. **c** Dialysis, end-stage renal disease. Code 90966 is for end-stage renal disease (ESRD)-related services for home dialysis per full month for patients 20 years and older (Smith 2012, 227).

64. **c** Code 97113, Therapeutic procedure, one or more areas, each 15 minutes of aquatic therapy with therapeutic exercises, is billable per 15 minutes of therapy. The patient was treated for 30 minutes; therefore, code 97113 should be reported twice. Modifier –50 is not applicable because the service is not a bilateral procedure (Smith 2012, 239).

65. **a** The *geometric mean LOS* is defined as the total days of service, excluding any outliers or transfers, divided by the total number of patients (Johns 2011, 323).

66. **b** Multiple surgical procedures with payment status indicator T performed during the same operative session are discounted. The highest-weighted procedure is fully reimbursed. All other procedures with payment status indicator T are reimbursed at 50% (Casto and Layman 2011, 183).

67. **c** Radiology procedures are identified under the outpatient perspective payment system with a status indicator X. Status indicator X identifies ancillary services that are separately paid (Johns 2011, 329–331).

68. **a** Psychiatric and rehabilitation hospitals, long-term care hospitals, children's hospitals, cancer hospitals, and critical access hospitals are paid on the basis of reasonable cost, subject to payment limits per discharge or under separate PPS (Johns 2011, 322).

69. **c** Diagnosis-related groupings (DRGs) are classified by one of 25 major diagnostic categories (MDCs) (Johns 2011, 322).

70. **d** Radiology procedures performed as outpatients are paid under the Medicare prospective payment system and are identified with a status indicator X for ancillary services (Johns 2011, 329–331).

71. **b** Critical access hospitals are paid on a cost-based payment system and are not part of the prospective payment system (Johns 2011, 330).

72. **a** Third-party payers who reimburse providers on a fee-for-service basis generally update fee schedules on an annual basis (Johns 2011, 350).

73. **a** Physicians submit claims via the electronic format (screen 837P), which takes the place of the CMS-1500 billing form (Johns 2011, 343).

74. **b** To accept assignment means the provider or supplier accepts, as payment in full, the allowed charge from the fee schedule (Johns 2011, 350).

75. **c** Review the elements of the hospital compliance program with the employee (Johns 2011, 361–362).

76. **b** Since 1983, the prospective payment systems have been used to manage the costs of the Medicare and Medicaid programs (Johns 2011, 287, 319).

77. **c** Access to an indwelling IV or insertion of a subcutaneous catheter or port for the purpose of a therapeutic infusion is considered part of the procedure and not separately billed (Smith 2012, 237).

78. **a** The goal of a compliance program is to prevent accusations of fraud and abuse (Johns 2011, 359).

79. **a** Any secondary diagnoses assigned present on admission status will have a negative impact on reimbursement if no other code on the claim is assigned as a complication or comorbidity or a major complication or comorbidity (Russo 2010, chapter 3).

80. **c** Payment for separately paid APCs depends on the status indicator assigned to each HCPCS code. This particular example allows separate payment on all five codes based on separately paid status indicator assignment (Johns 2011, 330–332).

81. **c** Out-of-pocket expenses are the healthcare expenses that the insured party is responsible for paying after the insurer has paid its amount. In the example, after the allowed charges of 80%, or $400, are covered by the insurance company, the patient will be responsible for the remaining 20%, or $100 (Johns 2011, 288, 316).

82. **a** Managed FFS reimbursement is similar to traditional FFS reimbursement except that managed care plans control costs primarily by managing their members' use of healthcare services (Johns 2011, 287, 316).

83. **d** The case-mix index is 1.45 for the total case-mix index of the hospital. An individual MS-DRG case mix can be figured by multiplying the relative weight of each MS-DRG by the number of discharges within that MS-DRG. This provides the total weight for each MS-DRG. The sum of all total weights (15,192) divided by the sum of total patient discharges (10,471) equals the case-mix index (Johns 2011, 324).

84. **d** Discounting applies to multiple surgical procedures furnished during the same operative session. The full rate will be paid to the surgical procedure with the highest rate and the additional procedures will be discounted 50% of their APC rate (Johns 2011, 330).

85. **c** An *appeal* is a request for consideration of denial of coverage for healthcare services of a claim (Casto and Layman 2011, 71).

86. **d** Prior approval for a service or procedure is called precertification and allows coverage for a specific service (Casto and Layman 2011, 71).

87. **d** Editing is not based on the clinical documentation of the discharge summary. Edits are predetermined based on coding conventions defined in the CPT codebooks, national and local policies and coding edits, analysis of standard medical and surgical practice, and review of current coding practices (Johns 2011, 347).

88. **a** Portions of the NCCI are incorporated into the outpatient code editor (OCE) against which all ambulatory claims are reviewed. The OCE also applies a set of logical rules to determine whether various combinations of codes are correct and appropriately represent services provided (Johns 2011, 348).

89. **c** Outpatient claims editor does not exist. Do not confuse this terminology with outpatient code editor (OCE) (Johns 2011, 348).

90. **b** Clean claims are essential for accurate and timely reimbursement (Casto and Layman 2011, 72).

91. **a** A patient name or certificate number is required for filing health claims (Casto and Layman 2011, 72).

92. **d** A procedure name is not a required element on a healthcare insurance claim (Casto and Layman 2011, 73).

93. **a** VBID calculates both the benefit and the costs of clinical services (Casto and Layman 2011, 77).

94. **a** The electronic format for institutional or facility claims is 837I for institutional claims, whereas 837P is for professional claims. The UB-04 and the 1500 forms are the paper billing forms for hospital (technical) and clinic (professional) claims, respectively (Casto and Layman 2011, 72).

95. **c** *Adjudication* is the determination of the reimbursement payment based on the member's insurance benefits (Casto and Layman 2011, 72).

96. **c** Claims that automatically process through computer software either auto-pay, auto-suspend, or auto-deny (Casto and Layman 2011, 72).

97. **b** Relative value units (RVUs) are assigned to each service to provide a value that correlates to payment (Casto and Layman 2011, 152).

98. **d** A service must not be solely for the convenience of the insured, the insured's family, or the provider (Casto and Layman 2011, 99).

99. **b** Coordination of benefits is necessary to determine which policy is primary and which is secondary so that there is no duplication of payments (Johns 2011, 343).

100. **b** A DRG is a predetermined amount of reimbursement for each Medicare inpatient (Johns 2011, 319).

101. **d** Medicare Part D pays for prescription drugs for beneficiaries (Hazelwood and Venable 2012, 324).

102. **c**   Medicaid is designed to offer assistance to low-income people and is jointly administered by the federal and state government (Hazelwood and Venable 2012, 327).

103. **a**   Conversion factor is a national dollar amount that Congress uses to convert relative value units to dollars on an annual basis (Hazelwood and Venable 2012, 331).

104. **b**   Discharges. The case-mix index can be figured by multiplying the relative weight of each MS-DRG by the number of discharges within that MS-DRG (Johns 2011, 324).

105. **b**   The payment varies based on the APC group (Johns 2011, 329).

106. **a**   The Healthcare Common Procedural Coding System (HCPCS) identifies and groups the services within each APC group (Johns 2011, 329).

107. **c**   The health information department along with the business office and cardiac department should be consulted to determine where the breakdown of the charges and assignment of the procedure code occurs. Often one department assumes another department is submitting the code or charge and without auditing and communicating with each other on a regular basis, error can occur for long periods of time with either a financial gain or loss to the facility (Casto and Layman 2011, 258).

108. **b**   Medicare administrative contractors (MACs) are replacing the claims payment contractors known as FIs and carriers (Casto and Layman 2011, 254).

109. **a**   HCPCS codes that are assigned in the charge description master that flow directly to the claim and bypass facility coding staff is a process known as hard coding (Casto and Layman 2011, 250).

110. **b**   The person responsible for the bill is the *guarantor* (Casto and Layman 2011, 8).

111. **c**   Clinical data document the patient's medical condition, diagnosis, and procedures performed as well as healthcare treatment provided (Johns 2011, 61).

112. **c**   The operative report includes a description of the procedure performed (Johns 2011, 73).

113. **a**   Results for lab tests will be included in a medical laboratory report (Johns 2011, 70).

114. **d**   Results of an x-ray interpretation by a radiologist are reported in a radiography report (Johns 2011, 70).

115. **c**   Results of the physician's examination of the patient's physical condition is reported in a physical examination report (Johns 2011, 63).

116. **b**   Pathological examinations of tissue samples and tissues or organs removed during surgical procedures are reported in the pathology report (Johns 2011, 77).

117. **a**   Physician orders are the instructions a physician gives to the other healthcare professionals. Admission and discharge orders should be found for every patient (Johns 2011, 63).

118. **c**   This information is collected by the examination of a newborn and reported on the newborn record (Johns 2011, 97).

119. **c** An ECG is a report of an electrocardiogram of the heart (Johns 2011, 70).

120. **b** A consultation report includes the recommendations of a consulting physician who is requested to evaluate a patient (Johns 2011, 78).

121. **d** After an initial assessment, documentation by other allied health professionals varies by specialty with appropriate content and frequency of recording (Johns 2011, 70).

122. **a** In 1974, the federal government adopted the UHDDS as the standard for collecting data for the Medicare and Medicaid programs. When the Prospective Payment Act was enacted in 1983, UHDDS definitions were incorporated into the rules and regulations for implementing diagnosis-related groups (DRGs). A key component was the incorporation of the definitions of principal diagnosis, principal procedure, and other significant procedures, into the DRG algorithms (LaTour and Eichenwald Maki 2010, 165).

123. **a** The ORYX Performance Measurement program collects quality data for hospitals and long-term care organizations and HEDIS collects data to measure physician performance (Johns 2011, 141).

124. **a** Subjective information includes symptoms and actions reported by the patient and not observed or measured by the healthcare provider (Johns 2011, 114).

125. **b** Objective information may be measured or observed by the healthcare provider (Johns 2011, 114).

126. **d** The plan includes orders and the roadmap for patient care (Johns 2011, 114).

127. **c** Professional conclusions reached from evaluation of the subjective or objective information make up the assessment (Johns 2011, 114).

128. **a** HIM professional analyze medical records for any missing reports, forms, or required signatures and deletions. This is a *quantitative analysis* of the medical record (Johns 2011, 409–410).

129. **c** Data currency and data timeliness refer to the requirement that healthcare data should be up-to-date and recorded at or near the time of the event or observation (Johns 2011, 48).

130. **b** Consistent data will be the same each time it is reported or collected (Johns 2011, 47).

131. **a** *Clinical data* document the patient's medical condition, diagnosis, and procedures performed as well as the healthcare treatment provided (Johns 2011, 61).

132. **a** Home health aides may assist the patient with activities of daily living such as bathing and housekeeping, which allows the patient to remain at home. Documentation of this type of intervention is also necessary (Johns 2011, 100).

133. **c** The emergency care record includes a pertinent history of the illness or injury and physical findings (Johns 2011, 93).

134. **d** The pathology report includes descriptions of the tissue from a gross or macroscopic level and representative cells at the microscopic level (Johns 2011, 77).

135. **d** The integrated health record is arranged so that the documentation from various sources is intermingled and follow strict chronological order (Johns 2011, 114).

136. **b** A complete medical history documents the patient's current complaints and symptoms and lists his and her past medical, personal, and family history (Johns 2011, 63).

137. **a** A physical examination report represents the attending physician's assessment of the patient's current health status (Johns 2011, 63).

138. **b** The consultation report documents the clinical opinion of a physician other than the primary or attending physician (Johns 2011, 78).

139. **c** Physician orders are the instructions the physician gives to the other healthcare professionals (Johns 2011, 63).

140. **a** *Hospice care* is palliative care provided to terminally ill patients and supportive services to patients and their families (Johns 2011, 101).

141. **a** In a joint effort of the Department of Health and Human Services (HHS), Office of Inspector General (OIG), Centers for Medicare and Medicaid Services (CMS), and Administration on Aging (AOA), Operation Restore Trust was released in 1995 to target fraud and abuse among healthcare providers (Casto and Layman 2011, 36).

142. **d** Tracking length of stay is part of the hospital utilization review committee function (Casto and Layman 2011, 42 and 46–47).

143. **c** Refiling claims after a denial is not possible because denied claims must be appealed and is not a factor in controlling fraud and abuse (Casto and Layman 2011, 35).

144. **b** Benchmarking or peer comparison helps a manager to know how his or her team has performed compared to peers. This includes whether the case-mix index level puts the facility at risk (Casto and Layman 2011, 43).

145. **d** The OIG workplan is published every year to provide insight into the directions the OIG is taking, as well as highlights of hot areas of compliance. Coding managers should review this document each year (Casto and Layman 2011, 43).

146. **b** The Voluntary Disclosure program was introduced in 1998 by the OIG to encourage healthcare providers to voluntarily report fraudulent conduct affecting federal payers (Johns 2011, 358).

147. **c** *Encryption* is the process of transforming text into an unintelligible string of characters that can be transmitted via communications media with a high degree of security and then decrypted when it reaches a secure destination (Johns 2011, 510).

148. **d** *Data reliability* is a method at looking at data quality consistently, sometimes referred to as data reliability. Reliability is frequently checked by having more than one person abstract data for the same case and compare the results for any discrepancies (Johns 2011, 509).

149. **c** HIPAA mandated incorporation of healthcare information standards into all electronic or computer-based health information systems (Johns 2011, 231).

150. **a** HL7 developed the HL7 Electronic Health Record System (EHR-S) Functional Model. It also includes many standards for data exchange with patient information (Johns 2011, 226).

151. **a** Pay for performance and pay for quality are types of incentive to improve clinical performance (Johns 2011, 154).

152. **b** Computer viruses and other malware constitute a threat to data security (Johns 2011, 510).

153. **b** Controlling access—facilities may authorize access to patient data in the facility's computer system to only those who need the access to do their job. This method of control serves the security of the data of patient records (Johns 2011, 510).

154. **b** An *audit trail* is a record of all transactions in the computer system, which is maintained and reviewed for instances of unauthorized access (Johns 2011, 510).

155. **c** HIM professionals have worked with many data stewardship issues for years (Johns 2011, 508).

156. **c** Be sure the employees receive appropriate compliance training and continue ongoing training for all employees (Johns 2011, 361–362).

157. **b** Establish a process, such as a hotline, to receive complaints and the adoption of procedures to protect the anonymity of complainants and to protect whistleblowers from retaliation (Johns 2011, 259).

158. **d** All newly hired coding personnel should receive extensive training on the facility's and HIM department's compliance programs. Education of the medical staff on documentation is likewise important to the success of any compliance program (Johns 2011, 362).

159. **d** The OIG continues to issue compliance program guidance since 1998 (Johns 2011, 359).

160. **c** *Upcoding* is the practice of assigning a diagnosis or procedure code specifically for the purpose of obtaining a higher level of payment (Johns 2011, 358).

161. **d** A *compliance officer* designs, implements, and maintains a compliance program that assures conformity to all types of regulatory and voluntary accreditation requirements governing the provision of healthcare products and services (Johns 2011, 744).

162. **b** *Concurrent review* occurs on a continuing basis during a patient's stay (Johns 2011, 410).

163. **a** Health Information Portability and Accountability Act of 1996 (Johns 2011, 692).

164. **d** An HIT professional must have knowledge of all the points addressed (Johns 2011, 801–804)

165. **c** The HIPAA Privacy Rule applies nationally to healthcare providers (Johns 2011, 801–804).

166. **d** Disclosures for which accounting is not required involve nine exceptions including those in the question (Johns 2011, 833).

167. **b** Notices of privacy must be posted in a prominent place where it is reasonable to expect that patients will read them (Johns 2011, 836).

168. **a.** An *incidental disclosure* occurs as part of a permitted use of disclosure (Johns 2011, 847).

169. **b** Data quality includes the following characteristics: accuracy, accessibility, comprehensiveness, consistency, currency, definition, granularity, precision, relevancy, and timeliness (Johns 2011, 43).

170. **b** *Data security* is the means of ensuring that data are kept safe from corruption and that access to data is suitably controlled (Johns 2011, 919).

171. **c** The type of tool used to aid in the coding process is called an encoder (Johns 2011, 269).

172. **d** A *portal* is a special application to provide secure remote access to specific applications (Johns 2011, 137).

173. **b** There are several different types of computer-assisted coding (CAC), including software to aid the physicians (Johns 2011, 270).

174. **b** *Natural-language processing* (NLP) is an artificial intelligence software that reads digital text from online documents and suggests codes to match the documentation (Johns 2011, 270).

175. **c** In an EHR, reports are indexed, similar to filing in the paper record, and ensure that the documents are placed in the right location within the right record. Record analysis and completion is done via computer. Document imaging converts paper documents into digitized electronic versions (Johns 2011, 432).

176. **d** The primary EHR applications include clinical documentation or patient care charting, computerized provider order entry, electronic medical administration records, and clinical decision support (Johns 2011, 137).

177. **a** *Data definition* means that the data and information documented in the health record are defined; users of the data must understand what the data mean and represent (Johns 2011, 48).

178. **b** Some encoders are built using expert system techniques such as rule-based systems, and other encoding software is more simplistic, merely automating a look-up function similar to the manual index in ICD or other coding classifications (Johns 2011, 269).

179. **a** Good encoding software should include edit checks to ensure data quality (Johns 2011, 270).

180. **c** A *unique patient identifier* is a unique number assigned by a healthcare provider to a patient that distinguishes the patient's medical records from all others (Johns 2011, 1178).

181. **b** One potential area for poor data quality surrounds the need for making data entry easier. These include "copy and paste," "macros," standard orders, and other techniques that "reuse" data. These techniques can make data entry faster, but care must be taken to ensure appropriate modification to the specific patient (Johns 2011, 182).

182. **b** For hospitals that do not have all EHR components, the result is a hybrid record that is part electronic and part paper. Some hospitals overcome hybrid record issues by scanning all paper documents into an EDMS, thereby making everything available online (Johns 2011, 148).

183. **b** Electronic signature authentication systems require the author to sign onto the system using a user ID and password, review the document to be signed, and indicate approval (Johns 2011, 144).

184. **d** In both the MS-DRG and APC groupings, coders enter the codes that have been selected in a computer program called a grouper. The grouper then assigns the patient's case to the correct group based on the ICD-9-CM and/or CPT/HCPCS codes (Johns 2011, 272).

185. **b** *Confidentiality* is a legal ethical concept that establishes the healthcare provider's responsibility for protecting health records and other personal and private information from unauthorized use or disclosure (Brodnik et al. 2009, 6).

186. **d** The UHCDA suggests that decision-making priority for an individual's next-of-kin be as follows: Spouse, adult child, parent, adult sibling, or if no one is available who is so related to the individual, authority may be granted to "an adult who exhibited special care and concern for the individual" (Brodnik et al. 2009, 113).

187. **b** A *subpoena* is a direct command that requires an individual or a representative of an organization to appear in court or to present an object to the court (Odom-Wesley et al. 2009, 57).

188. **a** The law permits a presumption of consent during emergency situations, regardless of whether the patient is an adult or a minor (Brodnik et al. 2009, 99).

189. **b** The Privacy Rule introduced the standard of minimum necessary to limit the amount of PHI used, disclosed, and requested. This means that healthcare providers and other covered entities must limit uses, disclosures, and requests to only the amount needed to accomplish the intended purpose (Johns 2011, 822).

190. **a** The HIPAA Privacy Rule provides patients with rights that allow them to have some control over their health information: right of access, right to request amendment of PHI, right to accounting of disclosures, right to request restrictions of PHI, right to request confidential communications, and right to complain of Privacy Rule violations (Johns 2011, 826).

191. **c** *Expressed consent* can be spoken or written (Johns 2011, 71).

192. **a** It is generally agreed that social security numbers (SSNs) should not be used as patient identifiers (Johns 2011, 387).

193. **b** Deidentified information is information that does not identify an individual; essentially it is information from which personal characteristics have been stripped (Johns 2011, 826).

194. **c** The notice of privacy includes a statement that the covered entity reserves the right to change the terms of its notice and to make the new notice provisions effective for all PHI that it maintains (Johns 2011, 837).

195. **a** Every member of the covered entity's workforce must be trained in PHI policies and procedures according to the Privacy Rule (Johns 2011, 857).

196. **c** *Subpoena duces tecum* is a written document directing individuals or organizations to furnish relevant documents and records (Johns 2011, 443; AHIMA 2012b, 329).

197. **c** A covered entity must act on an individual's request for review of PHI no later than 30 days after the request is made (Johns 2011, 831).

198. **a** The standard of minimum necessary means that healthcare providers and other covered entities must limit uses, disclosures, and requests to only the amount needed to accomplish the intended purpose (Johns 2011, 822).

199. **b** Under the Privacy Rule, healthcare providers are not required to obtain patient consent to use or disclose personally identifiable information for treatment, payment, or healthcare operations (Johns 2011, 838).

200. **b** The agreement between the covered entity and business associate should, at termination of the contract, require the business associate to return or destroy all PHI received from the covered entity that it still maintains and prohibit the associate from retaining it (Johns 2011, 824).

Practice Case Studies

Practice—Patient 1

PDX	550.90	Inguinal hernia, without mention of obstruction or gangrene, unilateral or unspecified (not specified as recurrent)
DX2	214.4	Lipoma of spermatic cord (as per path. and operative reports)
PP1	49505–LT	Repair initial inguinal hernia, age five years or older; reducible
PR2	55520–59	Excision of lesion of spermatic cord (separate procedure)

Notes for Practice Outpatient Case—Patient 1

550.90 The type of hernia is coded (Brown 2012, 208–209).

214.4 The lipoma is also removed and so should be coded (Brown 2012, 377–378).

49505–LT The hernia location is on the left and the laterality is reported (CPT Assistant September. 2000, 10).

55520–59 The lipoma requires excision and is therefore coded (CPT Assistant September. 2000, 10; October. 2001, 8).

(Garvin 2013, 48–52, 249.)

Practice—Patient 2

PDX	338.3	Neoplasm-related pain (acute) (chronic)
DX2	174.8	Malignant neoplasm of female breast, other specified sites
DX3	198.5	Secondary malignant neoplasm of bone and bone marrow
PP1	62362	Implantation or replacement of device for intrathecal or epidural drug infusion; programmable pump, including preparation of pump, with or without programming

Notes for Practice Outpatient Case—Patient 2

338.3   The patient is admitted for pain management due to metastatic cancer. If the admission is for pain control related to, associated with, or due to, a malignancy, code 338.3 (Brown 2012, 163; Coding Clinic 2nd Quarter 2007, 13–14).

174.8,   The primary site and metastatic (secondary) sites should be coded (Brown 2012, 378–382).

198.5

62362   The reservoir is surgically placed and attached to a previously placed catheter (CPT Assistant March 1997, 11).

(Garvin 2013, 54, 250.)

Practice—Patient 3

PDX	337.22	Reflex sympathetic dystrophy of the lower limb
PP1	64520–LT	Injection, anesthetic agent; lumbar or thoracic (paravertebral sympathetic)
PR2	77003	Fluoroscopic guidance and localization of needle or catheter tip for spine or paraspinous diagnostic or therapeutic injection procedures (epidural or subarachnoid)

Notes for Practice Outpatient Case—Patient 3

337.22   The diagnostic code is needed to establish the medical necessity for the procedure and a pain management code is not appropriate because the underlying condition is being treated (Brown 2012, 163).

64520–LT   When coding paravertebral spinal nerves and branches, it is appropriate to use the modifiers to note the laterality (CPT Assistant July 1998, 10; April 2005, 13).

77003   Fluoroscopic guidance is not included in the 64520 code; hence, it is therefore appropriate to code a second code (CPT Assistant March 2007, 7; July 2008, 9; February 2010, 12).

(Garvin 2013, 55, 251.)

Practice—Patient 4

PDX	038.42	Septicemia due to *Escherichia coli*
DX2	590.10	Acute pyelonephritis, without lesion of renal medullary necrosis
DX3	054.9	Herpes simplex without mention of complication
DX4	V09.0	Infection with microorganisms resistant to penicillins
DX5	305.1	Tobacco use disorder

Notes on Inpatient Practice Case—Patient 4

038.42   *E. coli* septicemia is documented on the culture and sensitivity as well as in the H & P. SIRS is not used here because septicemia is documented, versus sepsis (Brown 2012, 109–112).

590.10   Acute pyelonephritis is also coded because this is where the septicemia began. Do not code the organism (Coding Clinic 4th Quarter 1988). It is already reflected in the septicemia code (Brown 2012, 217).

054.9   Herpes simplex is documented on the 9/8 progress notes and is treated (Brown 2012, chapter 10).

305.1   Tobacco abuse is treated and documented in the progress notes, H & P and D/C summary. This code does not require a fifth digit (HHS 2011, Tabular Index; Brown 2012, chapter 12).

V09.0   The organism is specified to be resistant to in the discharge summary and therefore designate that in the coding (Brown 2012, 113).

Note: The pyelogram performed on 9/8 is not coded because it is an unspecified pyelogram (refer to the Procedures for Coding Medical Record Cases for the CCS Examination in the Introduction of this book). A pyelogram is coded only if it is code 87.74 or 87.76 (Retrogrades, urinary systems).

Points of Interest on Patient 4

1.   This case illustrates how an infection can begin in one organ system and then become systemic. This is why the same organism is in the urinary tract and the blood. As stated earlier, code both disorders (septicemia and pyelonephritis).

2.   The organism causing the infection is resistant to penicillin and ampicillin. Only code resistance to a drug if the resistance is documented by the practitioner in the record. Do not code from the laboratory reports alone.

(Garvin 2013, 68–75, 255.)

Practice—Patient 5

PDX	663.31	Delivery complicated by nuchal cord without compression
DX2	V27.0	Single liveborn
DX3	648.61	Other cardiovascular diseases in the mother classifiable elsewhere, but complicating pregnancy, childbirth, or the puerperium
DX4	424.0	Mitral valve disorders
PP1	73.6	Episiotomy

Notes on Inpatient 5

663.31 As per the delivery note, this is a delivery with a nuchal cord wrapped around the baby's neck (Brown 2012, 289).

V27.0 Outcome of delivery code (Brown 2012, 270).

648.61, These must be coded because they affected the monitoring of the patient and were documented in the medical record.

424.0 The "use additional code" note at category 648 directs the coder to add another code to identify the condition (Brown 2012, 276–277).

73.6 Episiotomy—the repair of an episiotomy is included in the code (Brown 2012, 282).

Points of Interest on Patient 5

1. In terms of documentation, this case is typical of many delivery charts. Often times, practitioners document the complication of delivery in only one area, such as the delivery note or the operative report. In this case, the baby has a nuchal cord, but it is only mentioned once in the delivery record.

2. This is also an illustration of the three types of codes, at a minimum, that must be on every delivery chart: a diagnostic code from the delivery or pregnancy category, an outcome of birth code (V code), and a procedure code.

(Garvin 2013, 124–126, 270.)

Practice —Patient 6

PDX	493.92	Asthma with (acute) exacerbation
PP1	99284–25	E/M code based on mapping scenario provided
PR2	96365	Intravenous infusion, for therapy, prophylaxis, or diagnosis (specify substance or drug); initial, up to one hour

Notes on Outpatient 6

493.92 This condition brought the patient to the emergency department (Brown 2012, 186–187).

99284–25 This code represents the evaluation and management code for the facility APV and is done according to the mapping scenario as follows; meds given are = 2 = 5 points, the history is problem focused = 10 points, the examination is extended problem focused = 15 points, the number of tests = 4 = 15 points, supplies = one venipuncture set and one intravenous set = 10 points. 55 total points.

96365   The IV infusion is separately reportable and an additional code should be assigned (CPT Changes: An Insider's View 2009).

Note: The patient came to the ED because of asthma. The code that represents the most complicated process is the evaluation and management of the patient represented by the E/M code and is sequenced first. The starting of the IV is less complicated and sequenced second.

(Garvin 2013, 193, 283.)

CCA Practice Exam 1

1. **d**   Index Fracture, femur, epiphysis, capital. Fifth digits are required for further classification of a specific condition. Many publishers include special symbols or color highlighting to identify codes that require a fourth or fifth digit (Schraffenberger 2012, 7).

2. **d**   Index Eruption, teeth/tooth, neonatal. Some main terms are followed by a list of indented subterms (modifiers) that affect the selection of an appropriate code for a given diagnosis. The subterms form individual line entries arranged in alphabetical order and printed in a regular type beginning with a lowercase letter. Subterms are indented on standard indention to the right under the main term. More specific subterms are further indented after the preceding subterm (Schraffenberger 2012, 12).

3. **a**   CPT code 21012 describes excision of a subcutaneous soft tissue tumor of the face or scalp greater than 2 cm and is appropriately coded when the tumor is removed from the subcutaneous tissue rather than subgaleal or intramuscular. Simple and intermediate closure of the wound is included in the procedure for the excision in the musculoskeletal section of CPT (AMA 2010, 28–29; AMA 2012, 88, 94–95).

4. **c**   Fine needle aspiration with image guidance is coded with 10022. Instructional note directs coder to assign 19295 for placement of localization clip during a breast biopsy. Add radiology code 76942 for supervision and interpretation of ultrasound guidance for localization clip guidance. See instructional notes following code 10022 (AMA 2012, 59).

5. **a**   Index Disease, Lou Gehrig's or Lou Gehrig's disease. Amyotrophic lateral sclerosis is another name for Lou Gehrig's disease. Many diseases carry the name of a person or an eponym. The main terms for eponyms are located in the Alphabetic Index under the eponym or the disease, syndrome, or disorder (Schraffenberger 2012, 13).

6. **d**   ICD-9-CM classifies cardiac pacemakers to code 37.8: Insertion, replacement, removal, and revision of pacemaker device. In coding initial insertion of a permanent pacemaker, two codes are required—one for the pacemaker (37.80–37.83) and one for the lead (37.70–37.74) (Schraffenberger 2012, 204–205).

7. **a**   When a pacemaker is replaced with another pacemaker, only the replaced pacemaker is coded (37.85–37.87). Removal of the old pacemaker is not coded (Schraffenberger 2012, 204–205).

8. **b** Index Block, left, with right bundle branch block. Right and left bundle branch block is inclusive of one code. It is inappropriate to assign a code for right (426.4) and left (426.3) bundle branch block when a combination code includes both the right and left (Schraffenberger 2012, 201–207).

9. **a** Index Fitting (of) pacemaker (cardiac). No procedure code exists in ICD-9-CM to describe reprogramming (Schraffenberger 2012, 204–205).

10. **d** SSS is the imprecise diagnosis with various characteristics treated with the insertion of a permanent cardiac pacemaker. The other three conditions are treated with cardioversion and different pharmacological therapy (Schraffenberger 2012, 194–195).

11. **c** Index Bypass, internal mammary-coronary artery (single), double vessel (36.16). Internal mammary-coronary artery bypass is accomplished by loosening the internal mammary artery from its normal position and using the internal mammary artery to bring blood from the subclavian artery to the occluded coronary artery. Codes are selected based on whether one or both internal mammary arteries are used, regardless of the number of coronary arteries involved (Schraffenberger 2012, 203–204).

12. **c** The Judkins technique provides x-ray imaging of the coronary arteries by introducing one catheter into the femoral artery with maneuvering up into the left coronary artery orifice, followed by a second catheter guided up into the right coronary artery, and subsequent injection of a contrast material (Schraffenberger 2012, 206).

13. **a** V58.83, encounter for therapeutic drug monitoring, is the correct code to use when a patient visit is for the sole purpose of undergoing a laboratory test to measure the drug level in the patient's blood or urine or to measure a specific function to assess the effectiveness of the drug. V58.83 may be used alone if the monitoring is for a drug that the patient is on for only a brief period, not long term. However, there is a Use Additional Code note after code V58.83 to remind the coder to use the additional code for any associated long-term drug use with codes V58.61–V58.69 (Schraffenberger 2012, 450–451).

14. **c** Code 43761 is assigned to report repositioning of a nasogastric or orogastric feeding tube through the duodenum. An instructional note guides the coder to report code 76000 when image guidance is performed (AMA 2012, 235).

15. **d** Code 49450 includes replacement of gastrostomy or cecostomy tube, percutaneous, under fluoroscopic guidance including contrast injections(s), image documentation, and report. Therefore, it would not be appropriate to add code 76000 for fluoroscopic guidance, which is already included in the procedure code (AMA 2012, 258).

16. **c** Index Ovum, blighted (Schraffenberger 2012, 282–283).

17. **b** Index Abortion, threatened 640.0. Refer to the ICD-9-CM Tabular List (640–649) for the correct fifth digit of 3, antepartum condition, not delivered (Schraffenberger 2012, 274–275).

18. **a** Index Delivery, cesarean, poor dilation, cervix (661.0). Refer to the ICD-9-CM Tabular (660–669) for the correct fifth digit of "1," delivered, with or without mention of antepartum condition. Outcome of delivery, single, liveborn. Cesarean section, low uterine segment (Schraffenberger 2012, 282–283).

19. **b** Index Rash, diaper. ICD-9-CM classifies dermatitis to categories 690–694. Atopic dermatitis and related conditions are specific to category 691. Fourth-digit subcategories include diaper or napkin rash and other atopic dermatitis and related conditions (Schraffenberger 2012, 292).

20. **a** Index Ingrowing, nail (finger) (toe) (infected) (Schraffenberger 2012, 295).

21. **b** Index Osteoarthrosis, localized, primary. For category 715, refer to the table for the fifth digit of 5 for pelvic region and thigh (Schraffenberger 2012, 303–304).

22. **a** Index Chondromalacia, patella (Schraffenberger 2012, 303–304).

23. **d** Index Paget's disease, bone. The main terms for eponyms are located in the Alphabetic Index under the eponym or the disease, syndrome, or disorder (Schraffenberger 2012, 13).

24. **d** Index Osteomyelitis, acute or subacute. Refer to the table in the Index for the fifth digit 5, ankle and foot. Infection, staphylococcal NEC (Schraffenberger 2012, 305–306).

25. **b** Index Anemia, aplastic, due to, antineoplastic chemotherapy. A coder should always assign the most specific type of anemia. Anemia due to chemotherapy is often aplastic (Schraffenberger 2012, 133–135).

26. **c** Index Exam, well baby. Premature, infant NEC. Refer to table in Tabular for fifth digit of "0" to note unspecified birth weight (Schraffenberger 2012, 324–328,).

27. **d** Index Dysfunction, diastolic (Schraffenberger 2012, 182–183).

28. **c** Use this code when the diagnosis is specified as a certain type of "benign mammary dysplasia," and in this case, "ductal" hyperplasia. Index Hyperplasia, breast, ductal, atypical (Schraffenberger 2012, 253).

29. **c** Index Bunionectomy or Mayo operation, bunionectomy. The main terms for eponyms are located in the Alphabetic Index under the eponym or the disease, syndrome, operation, or disorder (Schraffenberger 2012, 13).

30. **b** Index Lobectomy, lung, segmental (with resection of adjacent lobes), thoracoscopic. Segmental includes the complete excision of a lobe of the lung (Schraffenberger 2012, 227–228).

31. **d** Index Cholecystectomy (total), laparoscopic (Schraffenberger 2012, 237–238).

32. **c** Index Cystoscopy (transurethral), with biopsy (Schraffenberger 2012, 251).

33. **b** An *encoder* is a computer software program designed to assist coders in assigning appropriate clinical codes and helps ensure accurate reporting of diagnoses and procedures (LaTour and Eichenwald Maki 2010, 318–319).

34. **b** The RBRVS system is the federal government's payment system for physicians. It is a system of classifying health services based on the cost of furnishing physicians' services in different settings, the skill and training levels required to perform the services, and the time and risk involved (Casto and Layman 2011, 151).

35. **c** *Unbundling* is the practice of coding services separately that should be coded together as a package because all parts are included within one code and, therefore, one price. Unbundling, done deliberately, could be considered fraud (Kuehn 2012, 347).

36. **b** *CPT Assistant* provides additional CPT coding guidance on how to assign a CPT code by providing intent on the use of the code and explanation of parenthetical instructions. The American Medical Association publishes the guidance monthly (AMA 2012).

37. **b** *Unbundling* occurs when a panel code exists, and the individual tests are reported rather than the panel code (AMA 2012, 402).

38. **a** Reporting additional test codes that overlap codes in a panel allows the coder to assign all appropriate codes for services provided. It is inappropriate to assign additional panel codes when all codes in the panel are not performed. Reporting individual lab codes is appropriate when all codes in a panel have not been provided (AMA 2012, 402).

39. **a** The coder should assign the most comprehensive code to describe the entire procedure performed. When a code describes the entire service provided, the coder should not code each component separately. Assigning additional codes inherent to the main code would be a form of unbundling (Hazelwood and Venable 2012, 336).

40. **b** CMS developed the NCCI to control improper coding practices leading to inappropriate payments in Part B claims (CMS 2012a).

41. **c** AHA's *Coding Clinic for ICD-9-CM* is a quarterly publication of the Central Office on ICD-9-CM, which allows coders to submit a request for coding advice through the coding publication.

42. **b** CMS developed MUEs to prevent providers from billing units in excess and receiving inappropriate payments. This new editing was the result of the outpatient prospective payment system that pays providers passed on the HCPCS/CPT code and units. Payment is directly related to units for specified HCPCS/CPT codes assigned to an ambulatory payment classification (CMS 2012b).

43. **c** The documentation of the charges and itemized bill is not the responsibility of the physician (Smith 2012, 7–8).

44. **d** The identity of the patient's nearest relative and an emergency contact number are not relative to securing payment from the insurer. The encounter should include the date of the encounter and the identity of the observer (Smith 2012, 8).

45. **b** The hospital will receive the same reimbursement regardless of the length of stay (Casto and Layman 2011, 12).

46. **a** Higher relative weights link to higher payment rates (Casto and Layman 2011, 13).

47. **c** Home health resource groups (HHRGs) represent the classification system established for the prospective reimbursement of covered home care services to Medicare beneficiaries during a 60-day episode of care (Johns 2011, 334).

48. **c** The resource-based relative value scale (RBRVS) system was implemented by CMS in 1992 for physicians' services such as office visits covered under Medicare Part B. The system reimburses physicians according to a fee schedule based on predetermined values assigned to specific services (Johns 2011, 326).

49. **c** Major diagnostic categories (MDCs), of which there are 25. The principal diagnosis determines the MDC assignment (Johns 2011, 322).

50. **a** Children's hospitals are excluded from PPS because the PPS diagnosis-related groups do not accurately account for the resource costs for the types of patients treated (Johns 2011, 321).

51. **c** CMS identified *hospital-acquired conditions* (not present on admission) as "reasonably preventable," and hospitals do not receive additional payment for cases in which these cases are present (Johns 2011, 326).

52. **c** Gram-negative pneumonia (Johns 2011, 326).

53. **a** Stage I and II pressure ulcers are not considered hospital-acquired conditions but stage III and IV are (Johns 2011, 326).

54. **b** The electronic claim form (screen 837I) replaced the UB-04 (CMS 1450) paper billing form (Johns 2011, 343).

55. **b** An EOB is a statement sent by a third-party payer to the patient to explain the services provided (Johns 2011, 343).

56. **c** Uniform Ambulatory Care Data Set (Odom-Wesley et al. 2009, 310).

57. **c** *Vocabulary standards* establish common definitions for medical terms to encourage consistent descriptions of an individual's condition in the health record (Johns 2011, 227).

58. **a** The *consultation report* documents the clinical opinion of a physician other than the primary or attending physician. The report is based on the consulting physician's examination of the patient and a review of his or her health record (Johns 2011, 78).

59. **a** The *discharge summary* provides an overview of the entire medical encounter to ensure the continuity of future care by providing information to the patient's attending physician, referring physician, and any consulting physicians, to provide information to support the activities of the medical staff review committee and to provide concise information that can be used to answer information requests from authorized individuals or entities (Johns 2011, 78).

60. **a** The *discharge summary* is a concise account of the patient's illness, course of treatment, response to treatment, and condition at the time the patient is discharged (Johns 2011, 78).

61. **c** The nature and duration of the symptoms that caused the patient to seek medical attention as stated in the patient's own words (Odom-Wesley et al. 2009, 331).

62. **a** *Clinical information* is data related to the patient's diagnosis or treatment in a healthcare facility (Odom-Wesley et al. 2009, 55).

63. **d** Financial data include details about the patient's occupation, employer, and insurance coverage (Odom-Wesley et al. 2009, 42).

64. **c** The *Subjective, Objective, Assessment, Plan (SOAP)* notes are part of the problem-oriented medical records (POMR) approach most commonly used by physicians and other healthcare professionals. SOAP notes are intended to improve the quality and continuity of client services by enhancing communication among healthcare professionals (Odom-Wesley et al. 2009, 217).

65. **b** The Uniform Ambulatory Care Data Set (UACDS) includes data elements specific to ambulatory care, such as the reason for the encounter with the healthcare provider (LaTour and Eichenwald Maki 2010, 166).

66. **a** The transfer or referral form provides document communication between caregivers in multiple healthcare settings. It is important that a patient's treatment plan be consistent as the patient moves through the healthcare delivery system (Odom-Wesley et al. 2009, 131).

67. **c** According to the Joint Commission, except in emergency situations, every surgical patient's chart must include a report of a complete history and physical conducted no more than seven days before the surgery is to be performed (Odom-Wesley et al. 2009, 150).

68. **a** According to the Joint Commission, the physical examination must be completed within 24 hours of admission (Odom-Wesley et al. 2009, 353).

69. **b** An incomplete record not rectified within a specific number of days as indicated in the medical staff rules and regulations is considered to be delinquent (Johns 2011, 412).

70. **b** A complete medical history documents the patient's current complaints and symptoms and lists the patient's past medical, social, and family history (Johns 2011, 63).

71. **b** The benefit of concurrent review is that content or authentication issues can be identified at the time of patient care and rectified in a timely manner (Johns 2011, 410).

72. **c** The HIM manager may compare organizational data with external data from peer groups to determine best practices (Johns 2011, 609).

73. **d** Surveyors review the documentation of patient care services to determine whether the standards for care are being met (Johns 2011, 40).

74. **c** Participating organizations must follow the Medicare Conditions of Participation to receive federal funds from the Medicare program for services rendered (Johns 2011, 61).

75. **c** The total size of a removed lesion, including margins, is needed for accurate coding. This information is best provided in the operative report. The pathology report typically provides the specimen size rather than the size of the excised lesion. Because the specimen tends to shrink, this is not an accurate measurement (Kuehn 2012, 110–111).

76. **b** The pathology report describes specimens examined by the pathologist (Johns 2011, 77).

77. **d** It is not appropriate for the coder to assume the removal was done by either snare or hot biopsy forceps. The ablation code is only assigned when a lesion is completely destroyed and no specimen is retrieved. The coding professional must query the physician to assign the appropriate code (AHIMA 2012a, 607).

78. **d** The RAC demonstration uncovered $1.03 billion of improper payments, of which 96% were overpayments and 4% were underpayments (Casto and Layman 2011, 39).

79. **c** Seven elements are required as part of the basic elements of a corporate compliance program, and a medical staff appointee is not one of them (Johns 2011, 274).

80. **d** Quality improvement (QI) programs have been in place in hospitals for years and have been required by the Medicare or Medicaid programs and accreditation standards. QI programs have covered medical staff as well as nursing and other departments or processes (LaTour and Eichenwald Maki 2010, 33).

81. **b** Hospitals are encouraged but not required to follow the same work plan as the OIG. Hospitals should review the plan carefully and plan their compliance program around the target areas (Johns 2011, 275).

82. **a** The coder is not following established policies (Johns 2011, 265–267).

83. **c** Proper and timely documentation of all physician and other professional services must be obtained before billing. Facilities should not provide any financial incentive that may tempt a coder to code claims improperly such as upcoding to higher DRGs, which result in higher pay (Johns 20011, 275).

84. **c.** *Medical identity theft* occurs when someone uses a person's name and sometimes other parts of their identity without the victim's knowledge or consent to obtain medical services or goods (Johns 2011, 773).

85. **b** With an automated tracking system, it is easy to track how many records are charged out of the system, their location, and whether they have been returned on the due dates indicated (Johns 2011, 402).

86. **a** Audit trails can provide tracking information such as who accessed which records and for what purpose (Johns 2011, 403).

87. **a** Role-based access control (RBAC) is a control system in which access decisions are based on the roles of individual users as part of an organization (Brodnik et al. 2009, 211).

88. **a** Encoders come in two distinct categories: logic-based and automated codebook formats. A *logic-based encoder* prompts the user through a variety of questions and choices based on the clinical terminology entered. The coder selects the most accurate code for a service or condition (and any possible complications or comorbidities). An *automated codebook* provides screen views that resemble the actual format of the coding system (LaTour and Eichenwald Maki 2010, 269).

89. **d** EDI allows the transfer (incoming and outgoing) of information directly from one computer to another by using flexible, standard formats (Johns 2011, 348).

90. **c** A *software interface* is a computer program that allows different applications to communicate and exchange data (Johns 2011, 137).

91. **a** *Clinical decision support* includes providing documentation of clinical findings and procedures, active reminders about medication administration, suggestions for prescribing less expensive but equally effective drugs, protocols for certain health maintenance procedures, alerts that a duplicate lab test is being ordered, and countless other decision-making aids for all stakeholders in the care process (Johns 2011, 138).

92. **b** An HIE organization requires an identity-matching algorithm and record locator service (RLS). An identity-matching algorithm must be used by the HIE to identify any patient for whom data are to be exchanged. This algorithm uses sophisticated probability equations to identify patients. The RLS, then, is a process that seeks information about where a patient may have a health record available to the HIE organization (Johns 2011, 151).

93. **c** The designated record set includes health records that are used to make decisions about the individual (Johns 2011, 822).

94. **a** The covered entity must provide access to the personal health information in the form or format requested when it is readily producible in such form or format. When it is not readily producible in the form or format requested, it must be produced in a readable hard-copy form or such other form or format agreed upon by the covered entity and the individual (Johns 2011, 831).

95. **c** *Confidentiality* refers to the expectation that the personal information shared by an individual with a healthcare provider during the course of care will be used only for its intended purpose (Johns 2011, 49).

96. **c** Because federal regulations such as HIPAA and state laws govern the release of health record information, HIM department personnel must know what information needs to be included on the authorization for it to be considered valid (Johns 2011, 443).

97. **b** It is suggested that covered entities use PHI with certain specified direct identifiers removed as a guideline for disclosing only minimum necessary information while providing the amount needed to accomplish the intended purpose (Johns 2011, 822).

98. **b** *Privacy* is the right of an individual to be left alone. It includes freedom from observation or intrusion into one's private affairs and the right to maintain control over certain personal and health information (Johns 2011, 755).

99. **d** Data integrity services ensure the data are not altered as they are stored or transmitted electronically (Johns 2011, 184).

100. **d** Security measures not only provide for confidentiality, but data integrity and data availability—the CIA of security (Johns 2011, 184).

CCA Practice Exam 2

1. **c** The residual condition or nature of the late effect is sequenced first, followed by the cause of the late effect (Hazelwood and Venable 2012, 60–61).

2. **c** The residual condition or nature of the late effect is sequenced first, followed by the cause of the late effect. Late effect exceptions occur when the late effect code has been expanded at the fourth- and fifth-digit level to include the manifestations. In this case, only one code is necessary to describe both the residual condition and cause of the late effect (Hazelwood and Venable 2012, 62).

3. **a** Conditions that are integral to the disease process should not be assigned as additional codes. The nausea and vomiting are integral to the disease, gastroenteritis (Hazelwood and Venable 2012, 68).

4. **d**   Review Tabular List: Findings, abnormal, without diagnosis, prostate specific antigen (PSA), 790.93, or Elevation, prostate specific antigen (PSA), 790.93 (Hazelwood and Venable 2012, 69).

5. **b**   Near-syncope and nausea are both signs and symptoms and therefore not integral to the other. Both conditions should be coded (Hazelwood and Venable 2012, 71).

6. **d**   The Index may mislead the coder to a nonspecific code. In this example, when the coder references "Abnormal" and subheading "glucose," the coder is directed to code 790.29. The coder should always reference the Tabular List to verify the code. During verification, the coder will see the selection for code 790.22, which accurately describes the specific abnormal finding of glucose tolerance test (Hazelwood and Venable 2012, 74).

7. **c**   Pneumonia, unspecified, is assigned 486 in the Alphabetic Index. Cough is integral to pneumonia and should not be coded separately (Hazelwood and Venable 2012, 68–73).

8. **a**   Code signs and symptoms when a condition is *ruled out,* which means the condition has been proven not to exist. The code for seizures (780.39) is assigned when a more specific diagnosis cannot be made even after all the facts bearing on the case have been investigated (Hazelwood and Venable 2012, 68–73).

9. **c**   Index Incontinence, stress, male, NEC 788.32. Category 788.3x indicates incontinence of urine with the fifth digit specific to different types such as urge, stress, mixed, and others (Hazelwood and Venable 2012, 73).

10. **d**   Abdominal pain includes fifth digits to identify the specific parts of the abdomen affected. Nausea and vomiting is a category common to stomach upset. The fifth digits provide specificity. Nausea and vomiting are coded together with a combination code when both exist. Diarrhea usually is a symptom of some other disorder or of a more severe disease, in which case it should not be coded separately. It is often accompanied by vomiting and various other symptoms that should be coded when present. Because, in this case, a distinct disease is not available, all the symptoms should be coded (Hazelwood and Venable 2012, 73).

11. **a**   Parentheses enclose supplementary words or explanatory information that may or may not be present in the statement of a diagnosis or procedure. They do not affect the code number assigned in the case. Terms in parentheses are considered nonessential modifiers, and all three volumes of ICD-9-CM use them. Bronchiectasis (fusiform) (postinfectious) (recurrent) is an example of a diagnosis statement with nonessential modifiers noted with parentheses (Schraffenberger 2012, 26–28).

12. **b**   Index Infarction, myocardium, anterolateral (wall) with fifth digit for initial episode (Schraffenberger 2012, 26–28).

13. **d**   Only confirmed cases of HIV infection or illness are reported whether inpatient or outpatient. 042, Human immunodeficiency virus (HIV) disease. Patients with HIV-related illness should be coded to category 042, which includes AIDS, AIDS-like syndrome, AIDS-related complex, and symptomatic HIV infection (Hazelwood and Venable 2012, 89-90).

14. **b** Connecting words or connecting terms are subterms that indicate a relationship between the main term and an associated condition or etiology in the Alphabetic Index. The connecting term "due to" connects the organism *E. coli* to the urinary tract infection. The instructional note "Use additional code" is found in the Tabular List of ICD-9-CM. This notation indicates that use of an additional code may provide a more complete picture of the diagnosis or procedure. The additional code should always be assigned if the health record provides supportive documentation. Infection, urinary (tract) Tabular List—use additional code to identify organism. Infection, *Escherichia coli* (Schraffenberger 2012, 22–23, 79).

15. **b** When a patient is admitted for the purpose of radiotherapy, chemotherapy, or immunotherapy and develops a complication, such as uncontrolled nausea and vomiting or dehydration, the principal diagnosis is the admission for radiotherapy (V58.0), the admission for the antineoplastic chemotherapy (V58.11), or the admission for the antineoplastic immunotherapy (V58.12). Additional codes would include the cancer and the complication(s) (Hazelwood and Venable 2012, 103).

16. **c** The terms *metastatic to* and *direct extension to* are used for classifying secondary malignant neoplasms in ICD-9-CM. For example, cancer described as "metastatic to a specific site" is interpreted as a secondary neoplasm of that site. The colon (153.9) is the primary site, and the lung (197.0) is the secondary site (Hazelwood and Venable 2012, 109).

17. **a** 038.11, Septicemia, *Staphylococcus aureus,* and 995.91, Sepsis. The "Code first" note following code 995.91 directs the coder to assign the code for the underlying infection first (Schraffenberger 2012, 80–81).

18. **c** Diabetes (without complication) with fifth digit of 2 = type II, uncontrolled. 263.1 Malnutrition, mild, not stated as related to diabetes (Schraffenberger 2012, 122–124).

19. **d** 288.00, Fever, neutropenic. Instructional note states to use additional code for any associated fever (780.61) (Schraffenberger 2012, 137–139).

20. **a** CPT code 82270 describes a test for occult blood using feces source for the purpose of neoplasm screening with the use of three cards or single triple card for consecutive collection (AMA 2012, 417).

21. **b** New technology is addressed by the Category III codes (AHIMA 2012a, 584).

22. **b** Because a separate procedure is considered a part of, and integral to, another, larger procedure, it is not coded when performed as part of the more extensive procedure. See Surgery Guidelines. It may, however, be coded when it is not performed as part of another, larger service; therefore, answer "c" is not correct (AHIMA 2012a, 586).

23. **b** The AMA developed and maintains CPT. CMS developed and maintains HCPCS Level II codes (AHIMA 2012a, 586).

24. **c** Any physician may use the codes in any section of CPT (AHIMA 2012a, 587).

25. **d** See instructional notes preceding code 99217. In order to report these codes, the admission order must designate observation status. Whether the patient meets admission criteria or is admitted following surgery does not affect the observation code selection. If the patient is admitted and discharged on the same date, codes 99234–99236 are appropriate (AMA 2012, 13).

26. **b** Documentation of history of use of drugs, alcohol, and tobacco is considered part of the social history. The review of systems is a part of the history of present illness. See E/M Services Guidelines, instructions for selecting a level of E/M service, in the CPT manual (AMA 2011a, 4–7).

27. **c** Tissue transplanted from one individual to another of the same species but different genotype is called an *allograft* or *allogeneic graft* (AHIMA 2012a, 592–593).

28. **b** See definitions preceding code 17311 (Mohs micrographic technique) in CPT Professional Edition (AMA 2012, 79).

29. **a** The "with manipulation" code is used because the fracture was manipulated, even if the manipulation did not result in clinical anatomic alignment. See Musculoskeletal Guidelines, Definitions (AHIMA 2012a, 597).

30. **d** Index Incision and drainage, shoulder, bursa, resulting in code 23031 (AHIMA 2012a, 598).

31. **a** If the tip of the catheter is manipulated, it is a selective catheterization. In the case of a nonselective catheterization, the tip of the catheter remains in either the aorta or the artery that was originally entered (AHIMA 2012a, 604).

32. **c** The only vessel coded is the final vessel entered. See instructional note preceding code 36000. Intermediate steps along the way are not reported (AHIMA 2012a, 604).

33. **b** Diagnosis codes are often the primary reason for a service to be considered covered or denied by the insurance company. Local and national policies include diagnosis codes that are used in software edits to automatically deny or approve processed claims. Denied services can be appealed, and the record can be submitted to support medical necessity if the service fails the automated review (Schraffenberger 2012, 476).

34. **b** The NUBC was established with the goal of developing an acceptable, uniform bill that would consolidate the numerous billing forms hospitals were required to use (Schraffenberger 2012, 65).

35. **c** The Uniform Hospital Discharge Data Set was promulgated by the US Department of Health, Education, and Welfare in 1974 as a minimum, common core of data on individual acute-care, short-term hospital discharges in Medicare and Medicaid programs. It sought to improve the uniformity and comparability of hospital discharge data. In 1985, the data were expanded to include all nonoutpatient settings (Schraffenberger 2012, 63–65).

36. **a** For fiscal year 2008, Medicare adopted a severity-adjusted diagnosis-related groups system called Medicare Severity-DRGs (MS-DRGs). This was the most drastic revision to the DRG system in 24 years. The goal of the new MS-DRG system was to significantly improve Medicare's ability to recognize severity of illness in its inpatient hospital payments. The new system is projected to increase payments to hospitals for services provided to the sicker patients and decrease payments for treating less severely ill patients (Schraffenberger 2012, 471–473).

37. **a** For any given patient in a MS-DRG, the hospital knows, in advance, the amount of reimbursement it will receive from Medicare. It is the responsibility of the hospital to ensure that its resource use is in line with the payment (Schraffenberger 2012, 471–473).

38. **d**   Medicare provides for additional payment for other factors related to a particular hospital's business. If the hospital treats a high percentage of low-income patients, it receives a percentage add-on payment applied to the MS-DRG adjusted base payment rate. This add-on payment, known as the disproportionate share hospital (DSH) adjustment, provides for a percentage increase in Medicare payments to hospitals that qualify under either of two statutory formulas designed to identify hospitals that serve these areas. Hospitals that have approved teaching hospitals also receive a percentage add-on payment for each Medicare discharged paid under IPPS, known as the indirect medical education (IME) adjustment. The percentage varies, depending on the ratio of residents to beds. Additional payments are made for new technologies or medical services that have been approved for special add-on payments. Finally, the costs incurred by a hospital for a Medicare beneficiary are evaluated to determine whether the hospital is eligible for an additional payment as an outlier case. This additional payment is designed to protect the hospital from large financial losses due to unusually expensive cases (Schraffenberger 2012, 471–473).

39. **b**   Congress directed HHS to conduct a three-year demonstration project using RACs to detect and correct improper payments in the Medicare traditional fee-for-service program. Congress further required HHS to make the RAC program permanent and nationwide by January 1, 2010 (Schraffenberger 2012, 475).

40. **d**   Effective January 1, 2011, CMS allows a total of 25 ICD-9-CM procedure codes for 837 Institutional claims filing (Schraffenberger 2012, 66).

41. **b**   Attending and consulting physicians have no bearing on the assignment of the MS-DRG and payment to the hospital (Schraffenberger 2012, 471–473).

42. **b**   As of January 1, 2011, CMS allows a total of 25 ICD-9-CM diagnosis codes (1 principal and 24 additional diagnoses) for 837 Institutional claims filing (Schraffenberger 2012, 66).

43. **b**   Billing for two services that are prohibited from being billed on the same day. (Johns 2011, 347).

44. **c**   Remittance advice (RA) is sent to the provider to explain payments made by third-party payers (Johns 2011, 346).

45. **b**   The monies collected from third-party payers cannot be greater than the amount of the provider's charges (Johns 2011, 343).

46. **c**   Improve documentation to support services billed (Johns 2011, 348).

47. **c**   To qualify for a cost outlier, a hospital's charges for a case (adjusted to cost) must exceed the payment rate for the MS-DRG by a specific threshold amount determined by CMS for each fiscal year (Johns 2011, 374).

48. **c**   A *chargemaster* is a financial management form that contains information about the organization's charges for the healthcare services it provides to patients. Answer "a" is coinsurance. Answer "b" is budget. Answer "d" is expense (Johns 2011, 1116).

49. **a**   A *fee schedule* is a list of healthcare services and procedures and charges associated with each (Johns 2011, 350).

50. **b**   *Balance billing* means the patient cannot be held responsible for charges in excess of the Medicare fee schedule (Johns 2011, 350).

51. **a** An advance beneficiary notice (ABN) must be given to the patient to sign before treatment if any indication presents that may cause the service to be denied by Medicare (Johns 2011, 350).

52. **a** When a physician accepts assignment of benefits, the physician can only collect any applicable deductible or coinsurance from the patient (Casto and Layman 2011, 156).

53. **c** Budget neutrality must be maintained annually when the RVUs are adjusted (Casto and Layman 2011, 156).

54. **b** Generally, reimbursement for healthcare services is dependent on patients having health insurance (Casto and Layman 2011, 3).

55. **a** Health insurance for spouses, children, or both is known as dependent (family) coverage (Casto and Layman 2011, 5).

56. **b** A complete medical history documents the patient's current complaints and symptoms and lists his or her past medical, personal, and family history (Johns 2011, 63).

57. **a** *Present on admission* is defined as present at the time the order for inpatient admission occurs (CMS 2011c, 97).

58. **b** *Medical history* documents the patient's current complaints and symptoms and lists the patient's past medical, personal, and family history. The physical examination report represents the attending physician's assessment of the patient's current health status (Johns 2011, 63).

59. **a** An *operative report* describes the surgical procedures performed on the patient (Johns 2011, 73).

60. **d** The *physical examination report* represents the attending physician's assessment of the patient's current health status (Johns 2011, 63).

61. **c** A *pathology report* usually includes descriptions of the tissue from a gross or macroscopic level and representative cells at the microscopic level along with interpretive findings (Johns 2011, 77).

62. **c** The American College of Surgeons started its Hospital Standardization Program in 1918 (Johns 2011, 679).

63. **c** All entries must be legible and complete and must be authenticated and dated promptly by the person (identified by name and discipline) who is responsible for ordering, providing, or evaluating the service furnished (42 CFR 482.24).

64. **d** In a paper-based health record environment, corrections to health record entries are corrected by drawing a single line through the original entry, writing "error" above the entry, and then the practitioner signs, dates, and times the correction (Johns 2011, 413).

65. **c** Staff participation in the process of developing and implementing a program will contribute to the staff understanding of the importance of the program (Russo 2010, chapter 6).

66. **c** An addendum may be included in the medical record to update or supplement documentation that has been recorded (AHIMA 2008, 83–88).

67. **b** Documentation policies are used to define the acceptable practices that should be followed by all applicable staff to ensure consistency, continuity, and clarity in documentation (AHIMA 2005).

68. **d** In order to thoughtfully and appropriately manage copy functionality, organizations must have sound documentation integrity policies within their organization. HIM professionals should lead their organizations in developing copy policies and procedures that address operational processes, utilization of copy functionality, documentation guidelines, responsibility, and auditing and reporting (AHIMA 2012b, 9–10, 18–21). Documentation policies are used to define the acceptable practices that should be followed by all applicable staff to ensure consistency and continuity and clarity in documentation (AHIMA 2005).

69. **a** The physician principally responsible for the patient's hospital care writes and signs the discharge summary (Odom-Wesley et al. 2009, 200).

70. **a** *Histology* refers to the tissue type of a lesion. The histology of tissue is determined by a pathologist and documented in the pathology report (Johns 2011, 77).

71. **a** HIM ethical obligations apply regardless of employment site (Johns 2011, 754).

72. **a** *Privacy* is the right of an individual to be left alone (Johns 2011, 755).

73. **a** Corrective action should be taken when error or accuracy rates are deemed to be at an unacceptable rate (Johns 2011, 417).

74. **d** *Standards* are fixed rules that must be followed, which is different from a guideline that provides general direction (Johns 2011, 416).

75. **b** The system not recording who entered the data (Johns 2011, 433).

76. **d** The addendum must have a separate signature, date, and time from the original entry (Johns 2011, 437).

77. **a** An individual's right extends for as long as the record is maintained (Johns 2011, 827).

78. **c** HIPAA regulations preempt less strict state statutes where they exist (Johns 2011, 820).

79. **a** The Privacy Rule is applicable to all covered entities involved, either directly or indirectly, with transmitting or performing any electronic transactions specified in the act (Johns 2011, 823).

80. **d** Confidentiality is the responsibility for limiting disclosure (Johns 2011, 755).

81. **a** The Joint Commission, Commission on Accreditation of Rehabilitation Facilities, and the National Committee for Quality Assurance are all acceptable accrediting bodies for behavioral healthcare settings (Odom-Wesley et al. 2009, 447).

82. **b** *Identifier standards* establish methods for assigning a unique identifier to individual patients, healthcare professionals, healthcare provider organizations, and healthcare vendors and suppliers (Odom-Wesley et al. 2009, 311).

83. **c**   State licensure agencies have regulations that are modeled after the Medicare Conditions of Participation and Joint Commission standards. States conduct annual surveys to determine the hospital's continued compliance with licensure standards (Odom-Wesley et al. 2009, 287).

84. **b**   A *blanket authorization* is a common ethical problem when misused. Patients often sign a blanket authorization, which authorizes the release of information from that point forward, without understanding the implications. The problem is the patient is not aware of what information is being accessed (Johns 2011, 778–779).

85. **b**   Automatic session termination will help to control access to the computer when unattended by automatically ending the session when not in use, preventing unauthorized access (HHS 2006).

86. **c**   Edit checks help ensure data integrity by allowing only reasonable and predetermined values to be entered into the computer (Johns 2011, 509).

87. **b**   When several people enter data in an EHR, you can define how users must enter data in specific fields to help maintain consistency. For example, an input mask for a form means that users can only enter the date in a specified format (MacDonald 2007, chapter 4).

88. **c**   Automated systems for registering patients and tracking their encounters are commonly known as admission-discharge-transfer (ADT) systems (Johns 2011, 947).

89. **b**   A *data warehouse* is a special type of database that consolidates and stores data from various databases (Johns 2011, 909).

90. **b**   *Computer-assisted coding* is defined as the use of computer software that automatically generates a set of medical codes for review, validation, and use based on the documentation from the various providers of healthcare (AHIMA 2010b, 62; LaTour and Eichenwald Maki 2010, 400).

91. **a**   An *encoder* is computer software that helps the coding professional assign codes (Johns 2011, 269).

92. **c**   *Natural-language processing* (NLP) uses artificial intelligence software to allow digital text from online documents stored in the organization's information system to be read directly by the software, which then suggests codes to match the documentation (Johns 2011, 170).

93. **b**   All data security policies and procedures should be reviewed and evaluated at least every year to make sure they are up-to-date and still relevant to the organization (Johns 2011, 995).

94. **b**   *Beneficence* means promoting good (Johns 2011, 1113).

95. **b**   Threats to data security caused by people can be classified as threats from insiders who make unintentional mistakes, threats from insiders who abuse their access privileges to information, threats from insiders who access information or computer systems for spite or profit, threats from insiders who attempt to access information or steal physical resources, and from vengeful employees or outsiders who mount attacks on the organization's information systems (Johns 2011, 987).

96. **d**   The distinction of psychotherapy notes is important due to HIPAA requirements that these notes may not be released unless specifically specified in an authorization (Odom-Wesley et al. 2009, 440).

97. **d** When a person or entity willfully and knowingly violates the HIPAA Privacy Rule, a fine of not more than $250,000, not more than 10 years in jail, or both may be imposed (LaTour and Eichenwald Maki 2010, 292).

98. **d** *Access control* means being able to identify which employees should have access to what data (Johns 2011, 992).

99. **b** An EHR can be viewed by multiple users and from multiple locations at any time, and organizations must have in place appropriate security access control measures to ensure the safety of the data (Johns 2011, 435).

100. **c** When a state law is more stringent than a federal law, hospitals must comply with both (Odom-Wesley et al. 2009, 68).

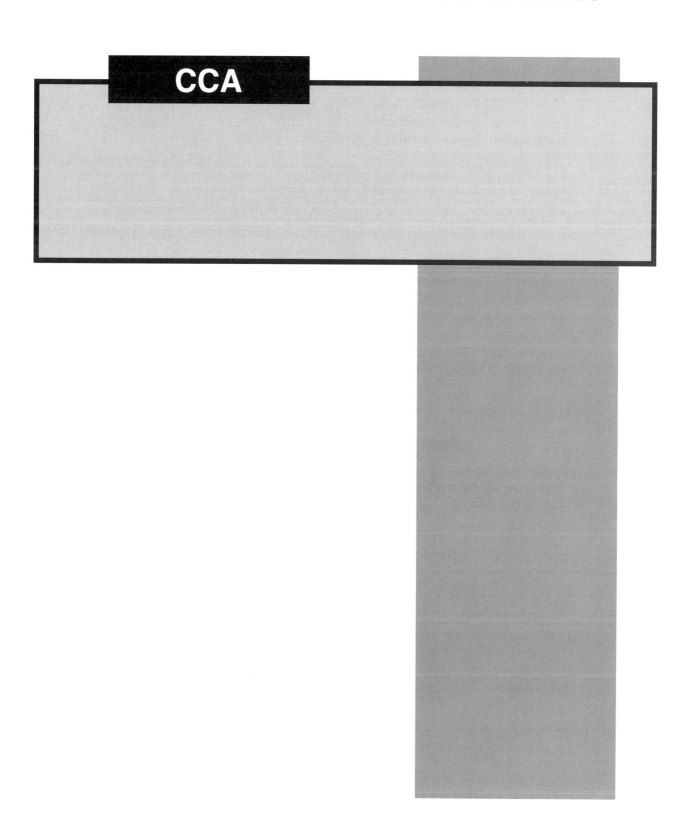

References

CCA

References

42 CFR 482.24: Medical Record Services. 2010.

American Health Information Management Association. 2012a. *Clinical Coding Workout: Practice Exercises for Skill Development with Answers.* 2012 ed. Chicago. AHIMA.

American Health Information Management Association. 2012b. *Copy Functionality Toolkit.* Chicago. AHIMA.

American Health Information Management Association. 2012c. *Pocket Glossary of Health Information Management and Technology.* 3rd ed. Chicago: AHIMA.

American Health Information Management Association. 2008. Practice brief: Managing an effective query process. *Journal of AHIMA,* 79(10). Chicago: AHIMA.

American Health Information Management Association. 2005. e-HIM Work Group on Maintaining the Legal EHR. Update: Maintaining a legally sound health record—Paper and electronic. *Journal of AHIMA* 76(10): 64A–L. Chicago: AHIMA.

American Hospital Association. *Coding Clinic for ICD-9-CM* 2009, 1Q:20. Chicago: AHA.

American Hospital Association. *Coding Clinic for ICD-9-CM* 2004, 3Q:4. Chicago: AHA.

American Hospital Association. *Coding Clinic for ICD-9-CM* 2000, 3Q:6 Chicago: AHA.

American Hospital Association. *Coding Clinic for ICD-9-CM* 1992, 2Q:15–16. Chicago: AHA.

American Medical Association. 2012. *CPT Current Procedural Terminology. Professional Edition.* Chicago: AMA.

American Medical Association. 2010. *CPT Current Procedural Terminology Changes: An Insider's View.* Chicago: AMA.

Brodnik, M., M. McCain, L., Rinehart-Thompson, and R. Reynolds. 2009 *Fundamentals of Law for Health Informatics and Information Management,* Chicago: AHIMA.

Casto, A. and E. Layman. 2011. *Principles of Healthcare Reimbursement,* 3rd ed. Chicago: AHIMA.

Centers of Medicare and Medicaid. 2012a. National Correct Coding Initiative Edits. http://www.cms.gov/Medicare/Coding/NationalCorrectCodInitEd/index.html?redirect=/nationalcorrectcodinited/.

Centers of Medicare and Medicaid. 2012b. National Correct Coding Initiative, Medically Unlikely Edits http://www.cms.hhs.gov/NationalCorrectCodInitEd/08_MUE.asp#TopOfPage.

Centers for Medicare and Medicaid Services and the National Center for Health Statistics. 2011c. ICD-9-CM Official Guidelines for Coding and Reporting. http://www.cdc.gov/nchs/data/icd9/icd9cm_guidelines_2011.pdf.

Centers of Medicare and Medicaid. 2010a (February). http://www.cms.hhs.gov/MLNMattersArticles/downloads/MM6563.pdf.

Centers of Medicare and Medicaid. 2010b (February). http://www.cms.hhs.gov/ContractorLearningResources/downloads/JA6563.pdf.

Department of Health and Human Services. 2006. *HIPAA Security Guidance.* http://www.hhs.gov/ocr/privacy/hipaa/administrative/securityrule/remoteuse.pdf.

Hazelwood, A. and C. Venable. 2012. *ICD-9-CM and ICD-10-CM Diagnostic Coding and Reimbursement for Physician Services.* Chicago: AHIMA.

Johns, M.L., ed. 2011. *Health Information Management Technology: An Applied Approach,* 3rd ed. Chicago: AHIMA.

Joint Commission. (revised) 2009 (March). The Official Do Not Use List (April 2005). http://www
.jointcommission.org/Do_Not_Use_List_of_Abbreviations/ and http://www.jointcommission.org/
facts_about_the_official_%E2%80%9Cdo_not_use%E2%80%9D_list/. Oakbrook Terrace, IL: The
Joint Commission.

Kuehn, L. 2012. *Procedural Coding and Reimbursement for Physician Services: Applying Current
Procedural Terminology and HCPCS.* Chicago: AHIMA.

LaTour, K. and S. Eichenwald Maki, eds. 2010. *Health Information Management: Concepts, Principles,
and Practice,* 3rd ed. Chicago: AHIMA.

MacDonald, M. 2007. *Access 2007: The Missing Manual.* Sebastopol, CA: O'Reilly Media, Inc.

Odom-Wesley, B., D. Brown, and C. Meyers. 2009. *Documentation for Medical Records.* Chicago:
AHIMA.

Pozgar, G.D. 2009. *Legal Essentials of Health Care Administration.* Sudbury, MA: Jones and Bartlett.

Russo, R. 2010. *Clinical Documentation Improvement: Achieving Excellence.* Chicago: AHIMA.

Sayles, N. and K. Trawick. 2010. *Introduction to Computer Systems for Health Information Technology.*
Chicago: AHIMA.

Schraffenberger, L.A. 2012. *Basic ICD-10-CM/PCS and ICD-9-CM Coding,* Chicago: AHIMA.

Smith, G. 2012. *Basic Current Procedural Terminology and HCPCS Coding.* Chicago: AHIMA.